P9-CKE-757

THE
Honest
Truth
ABOUT
Losing
Weight
AND
Keeping
It Off

THE
Honest Truth
ABOUT
Losing Weight
AND
Keeping It Off

Best "B healtth! Joan Price

JOAN PRICE, M.A.

NORDIC PRESS
MINNEAPOLIS
MINNESOTA

Copyright © 1991 NordicPress Books. All rights reserved. No part of this publication may be reproduced without written permission from the publisher.

Notice: The information and ideas in this book are for educational purposes and are not intended as prescriptive advice. Consult your physician before starting any exercise or weight loss program.

Library of Congress Catalog Card Number: 90-064113

ISBN: 0-9627708-1-7

Printed in the United States of America

91 92 93 94 95 96 / 6 5 4 3 2 1

NordicPress Books are available at quantity discounts with bulk purchase for educational, business, or sales promotional use. For information write:

Special Sales Department
NordicPress
141 Jonathan Boulevard North
Chaska, Minnesota 55318

Table of Contents

Foreword

American's perennial quest for thinner, more youthful figures has unfortunately brought with it an often bewildering array of faddish diets and bizarre weight loss schemes. Refreshingly, there's a fundamental change taking place in the way Americans try to lose weight. Fortunately, the trend is away from the oddly eccentric diet plans to the natural way of losing weight through exercise and more nutritious eating.

Joan Price's *The Honest Truth About Losing Weight And Keeping It Off* will not be your magic pill or quick fix gimmick, but it is an important part of this wholesome revolution. Price is an experienced writer on health-care issues and a tireless advocate for sensible weight-loss programs that emphasize exercise and low-fat eating as a sound way to permanently lose weight. If you're looking for a positive, well-balanced program to help you lose weight, you'll find this book is an effective tool.

Based on the latest research in the field of weight control, author Price provides an insightful analysis of what works for dieters and what doesn't. Price says the "honest truth" is that a low-fat food plan accompanied by a serious program of exercise can be your ticket to losing weight permanently. And it's a position that is gaining considerable headway against what sometimes seems a torrent of misinformation.

Price first presents a surprisingly candid review of the important diet books, programs, foods, and clubs for the overweight. Then, she teaches how to control hidden fats in your diet and increase complex carbohydrates.

Careful to recognize that Americans have widely varying tastes and eating lifestyles, her hope is to make you the expert so you can intelligently sift through the mountains of conflicting plans and programs to find the one that best suits your lifestyle.

Price also tackles the "truth about exercise." Her premise is both sound and unequivocal: a balanced exercise program that includes both strength training and aerobic exercise, is the surest, most effective way to lose weight and stay trim.

Price, an IDEA Foundation certified exercise instructor, provides a useful and stimulating section on motivation that is especially welcome, along with the log pages for noting the personal progress that almost surely will follow.

The Honest Truth About Losing Weight And Keeping It Off is important reading for:

Overweight readers who want to lose weight and open their lives to exhilarating new vistas of opportunity.

Health-conscious readers will discover easy-to-use techniques for reducing the amount of excess fat they eat.

Fitness-conscious Americans will find Price's techniques powerful incentives to starting and sticking to a lifelong program of exercise and healthy lifestyle.

Balance, variety, and moderation are all important guidelines stressed by Price, who promotes sound nutrition for promoting safe weight loss.

One word of advice: as you read this book, treat it like the high spirited adventure it is. It will go a long way toward helping you identify and direct positive energy toward reducing your weight and rejuvenating your quality of life.

Peg Connelly, R.N.
Nurse Director
Yale University Weight Control Program

Introduction

No More Empty Promises!

The Honest Truth About Losing Weight and Keeping It Off was written for those of you who want to make a permanent change in the shape, health and vigor of your body. If you really want to make changes, we promise to tell you the truth about how to make that happen.

We wrote this book because the dieting marketplace is glutted with all manner of books, pills, potions, and programs that purport to tell you the "truth" about losing weight.

But "truth" seems to come in various degrees these days. Hence, our less than grammatically perfect title which emphasizes the honest truth.

In this book, you're going to get the facts about what really works. We're not selling gimmicks. We're not selling fads or fancies. We're not going to ask you to give up food, put drops on your tongue, wear cellophane pants, or send for a month's supply of fat-burning pills. We have something much more substantial in mind. The plain, unvarnished truth.

If you don't know the truth about how to lose weight permanently, you'll learn it here. If you do know, we'll give you plenty of tips and nudges for creating an action plan to get started.

- You'll learn about the contemporary weight loss plans and programs and how to intelligently make good sense out of their claims and promises.

- You'll understand how your body responds to different methods of losing weight.
- You'll learn crucial facts about fat and how to lose it.
- You'll learn about how to choose a lifelong eating plan and lose that excess body fat.
- You'll learn how to use a balanced program of aerobic and strength training exercises to help you lose fat and keep it off permanently.
- You'll set personally meaningful goals that are realistic and achievable.
- Finally, you'll discover how to build the motivation you need to turn talk into action. You'll make changes that will help you lose excess body fat, become strong and lean, and improve your health, self-esteem, vitality, and quality of life.

Guess what? You've already started. By reading this book you've taken the first step. You're already involved in the process that will help you get and keep your body fat low—for life. You've taken the first step toward success.

Now, let's get the honest truth!

Part I

The Honest Truth

About Dieting

And

Permanent Weight Loss

1

Why Another
Diet Book?

How to write a best-selling diet book:

As a general rule of thumb, the diet should be as unnatural and unbalanced as possible; there is, by now, no other way to make it seem special.

—William Bennett, M.D. and Joel Gurin, in *The Dieter's Dilemma: Eating Less and Weighing More*, 1982, Basic Books

You stare at yourself in the mirror. You turn this way and that, but all you see are those bulges, folds and unsightly puckers.

You stand on the scale. Maybe if you exhaled all your breath . . . Maybe if you removed your watch . . . your ring.

Enough. You could paint these word pictures of yourself *ad infinitum*, remembering the last encounter with your scale, a mirror, or a swimsuit.

The fact is, you're altogether too familiar with the extent of your past caloric sins. What you need now is someone to help you get out of this mess. Perhaps, just one more diet. And let's face it, there are some loony diet books out there. Eat only fruit (*The Beverly Hills Diet*) . . . eat only rice (*The Rice Diet Report*) . . . don't mix carbohydrates and proteins (*Fit for Life*) . . . eat 600 calories for three days, then 900 calories for four days, then 1200 calories for a week (*The Rotation Diet*).

Not a shred of medical or nutritional evidence supports any of these claims. And yet these diets and thousands of others like them have been swallowed by an overweight populace eager for easy answers.

Sure, some of the diets you've tried produced weight loss. You can lose weight eating only cornbread, lizards or cardboard, for that matter. You can lose weight combining okra and oatmeal. It isn't the food, the food combination, or any alleged fat-burning qualities of those foods that produces weight loss.

Magic Pills, Potions, Doodads, And Other Miracles

You have only to read the ads in popular newspapers to become a believer in P.T. Barnum:

> **Do you want to LOSE 10, 15, even 25 lbs. IN JUST ONE WEEK without starving & exercising?** A proven European formula has been helping Americans lose weight successfully for 3 years—OVER 250,000 ORDERED.

Another shouts:

> **UNEXPLAINED WEIGHT LOSS PUZZLES SCIENTISTS** While it is not entirely clear how the formula induces weight loss, some scientists believe

> this compound actually alters the way the body digests food: when taken before mealtime it bonds with food and suppresses calorie absorption.

Or how about losing weight with Con Ed?

> **ELECTRIC VIBRATOR—FAT MELTS AWAY**. Just strap on to massage wherever you'd like to slim down: tummy, rear, hips, thighs. You can go about your business or just relax while the Electric Vibrator Belt does the hard work for you.

Perhaps you want to make unsightly cellulite vanish as easily as applying another new scientific breakthrough:

> **AMAZING NEW DISCOVERY ELIMINATES CELLULITE QUICKLY**. This amazing product is guaranteed to work or you (sic) money back. Apply generously to a (sic) affected areas. Work in well until a (sic) absorbed, then wrap with hot damp towels for 20 minutes . . . Harmful only if swallowed.

No, we're not making these up, and we didn't have to scour only the tabloids to find them. These are actual ads in a diet magazine that this author received unsolicited in the mail last month. It also advertises a metabolic booster ("so you can enjoy a normal and unhindered food intake and at the same time accomplish safe, effective and virtually automatic weight loss"), a "miracle soup diet" (Ms. R.S. from Little Rock lost 30 pounds in 2 weeks), and a dieter's pledge that includes "I will not expect help from others."

Wouldn't it be nice? We could lounge on the sofa, one hand reaching for chocolate creams and the other guiding the fat-melting vibrator to strategic spots on our bellies and thighs. We could pop a calorie-blocker an hour before our ice cream sundaes.

Sorry, folks, there's no miracle way to block, burn, rub, jiggle, vacuum, melt or wrap fat off our bodies. There's no magic pill, injection, cream, or potion. If there were, don't you think it would make the front page of all the newspapers and medical journals instead of being buried in a magazine of questionable repute?

Some of the more ridiculous weight loss gizmos of the past included special pants that attached to your vacuum cleaner to suck out fat and appetite-suppressing eyeglasses. Many of these gimmicks are relatively harmless, except, of course, to the buyer's dreams or wallet. However, one mail-order capsule which promised fast weight loss actually accomplished just that—it contained a tapeworm which eventually had to be surgically removed. Be wary. Be informed. People actually die from some of the remedies these quacks propose. The false-hope pushers are hungry for people so desperate to lose weight that they fall for these gimmicks. Don't be one of those people.

Each year, millions of Americans grimly renew the search for the holy grail of permanent slimness with this willful pledge: "This time, I'll do it!" They fill refrigerators with diet foods, join a health club, sign up with a weight loss support group, load up on calorie counters.

But ever present for almost all of those facing the melancholy prospect of paring unwanted pounds from bloated physiques is this dismal prognosis: fat chance.

Dieting Snapshots

• Ruth, 53, is always on a diet. "My daughter asks me, 'Mom, how many diets have you been on?' I tell her, 'All of them.' You name it, I've tried it. Don't they work? Oh yeah, they work. Until I stop. Do I have to spend the rest of my life dieting?"

• Sandra, 44, has clothing in three sizes in her closet. "I'm an expert at losing weight," she says lightly, but her smile fades quickly. "When my doctor says I should lose some weight, I tell her, 'Hey, I've lost 160 pounds!' And I have: 40 pounds, four times."

• Mike, 38, never gave a thought to his weight until recently. "I know I weigh a few pounds more than I did in college," he says with a laugh, "but I never worried about it until my seven-year-old daughter asked if my waist had 'slipped' because I was wearing my belt so low! I took a hard look at myself in the mirror, and I didn't like what I saw."

• Mary, 58, has tried every weight loss book on the market (and several now out of print). Her bookcase resembles the diet section of the public library. If there was a Diet-Book-of-the-Month Club, she would join.

Sixty stubborn pounds envelope her figure, a fatty wardrobe she hasn't changed substantially for 25 years. Though she always loses weight when she starts a new diet, she inevitably regains it as soon as she starts "eating" again. She recently announced, "I've figured out the ideal diet for me. From now on, I'm going to eat only foods I hate."

• Julie, 26, has been overweight all her life. "I was a fat baby, a fat kid, a fat teenager, and now I'm a fat adult. My whole family is fat. I know I'll never be skinny, and I'm not willing to starve myself to try. But my dad died young of heart disease, and my mother has diabetes. I'm worried about my health and I'm confused by everything I read. Don't eat *this*, eat *that*. Exercise *this* way, not *that*. Please, would someone just tell me the truth?"

The Problems With Diets

The problem here is this: reducing calories is only part of the solution. You can't stay on a low calorie diet forever.

Sooner or later, you've got to go back to real meals.

Most weight loss programs or restrictive diets don't prepare you for eating real food in the real world again. You're either on the diet (depriving yourself of food) or off the diet (eating the foods that put the weight on in the first place).

You lose weight on just about any diet because you're also restricting your calories, even when you don't intend to or realize it. And when you start eating regularly again, you're ravenous. It's like busting out of jail. Or a bear coming out of hibernation. You want to eat everything in sight—and most of what's hidden in the cupboards and grocer's freezer. You can't help yourself!

No, this isn't lack of willpower—it's your biological survival drive, ensuring that you'll put on some extra padding so you won't starve the next time food is scarce. And your slower metabolic rate lets the pounds come back quickly. We'll talk more about that later.

Do you see why extreme diets are temporary, unpleasant, nutritionally unsound, and destructive to your health? Worst of all, they don't even work.

You're Ready For Some Real Answers

You're tired of the amount of time and energy going into your weight. You're tired of denying yourself new clothes until you get to your goal size. And you're sick and tired of those diets, those *awful* diets.

You're ready for the last weight loss book you'll ever need, which gives facts, not fads. You want the honest truth about weight loss, nutrition and exercise, so you don't have to keep trying new weird diets or depriving yourself with rigid menus.

No Mystery, No Big Bucks

Weight loss is not a mysterious issue. You can learn the facts and understand how to make them work for you in the time it takes to read this book.

The truth about losing fat isn't complicated. It isn't a well-guarded secret. It isn't expensive. The annual cost will be no more than the price of this book; a year's worth of healthful, varied, nutritious foods; and perhaps a good piece of in-home exercise equipment to help you put your fitness plan into action.

Here's the straight, unvarnished truth:

1. There's no magic in eating some food with or without another, or eating at a certain time of day, or week, or month. No food or combination of food speeds up fat-burning—only exercise does that.
2. Those weird diets you've been using are nutritionally unbalanced and therefore far from healthful; you might be risking more than your pounds. Those diets make best-sellers, not best bodies.
3. You'll likely find that crazy diets will make you fatter and less healthy than when you started.

The honest truth is, losing weight permanently is easy. You need only two things:

1. A permanent exercise program that you enjoy
2. A few crucial changes in your eating behavior

Now, what could be simpler than that? That's why you're reading this book. You're not satisfied with the results of past dieting attempts. This time you're looking for something different. You want information, good hard facts. You want to understand, once and for all, what you have to do to lose weight permanently. You want a personalized action plan that will get you to your goals. You want to get going, lose the weight, and get on with your life.

How Is This Book Different?

First of all, it's not a diet book. It won't list untouchable foods. It will teach you to count fat instead of calories. You'll learn how to halt that cyclical pattern of losing and regaining weight—the yo-yo dieting that's not only hazardous to your health, but actually prevents you from making the weight loss progress that has been so elusive to you.

You'll learn the importance of exercise in speeding up your metabolism and increasing fat-burning lean tissue while decreasing fat tissue. You'll learn more about this exciting prospect in later chapters.

Best of all, your efforts will help you achieve balanced fitness and enhance the quality of your life. You'll feel different immediately.

This book will give you the information and skills to:

- Feel empowered, not deprived
- Feel in control, armed with information
- Learn about your own body: what it needs, why it seems to fight you when you diet, how to be its partner in health and well-being
- Choose the physical activity that keeps your body fat low and your self-esteem high
- Make changes in your eating and exercise habits to lose body fat gradually, safely, and permanently

- Develop a leaner look and have more energy
- Motivate yourself to make healthful habits a central part of your life

How Amy Successfully Used This Plan

Amy, 39, has been losing and gaining the same 5-20 pounds since high school. Though she's within the average weight range for her height, she's sure she would look and feel better if she could get rid of those few pounds forever.

Amy started on her weight loss roller coaster in college. She went to therapists, weight loss groups, a herbalist and a diet nutritionist. She tried liquid protein, coffee enemas, and every low-calorie diet she could find. She has a suitcase full of food diaries.

When she looks back at old pictures, Amy realizes, "I really didn't look so bad. But in high school, even if you were only 10 pounds overweight, the popular people were 10 pounds underweight. They had these model figures. Even if I was normal, everybody else seemed svelte. So in contrast, I looked that much bigger."

Now Amy exercises regularly and eats nutritious meals that are low in fat, low in sugar. And it wasn't hard at all, once her spirit of adventure took hold. Just take it a step at a time, and you'll be able to forget about dieting forever! It can work the same way for you. Here's how you'll do it!

First, in Part I of this book, you'll learn the Honest Truth about dieting. You'll discover what happens to your body when you diet; the crucial role of dietary fat in losing weight; which diet plans and programs will fit your eating lifestyle; and finally, how to make a smart, lifelong choice for eating more nutritiously, more enjoyably, and more in keeping with your long-term weight loss goals.

Part II will show you how a balanced exercise program including both aerobic exercise and strength training is just the ticket you need to pare pound after pound from your figure because it alters your body composition and your metabolic rate. You'll learn all the facts you need from the experts who know, including the folks at The National Exercise For Life Institute, which makes gathering and disseminating research on the benefits of exercise their one and only goal.

But knowing the vital secrets about eating right and getting exercise aren't enough. You need *motivation* to start and stick with these all-important plans, in order to turn talk into action.

That's what you'll find in Part III. You'll also find log pages to chart your progress to become simply the best you that you can be.

Now It's Your Turn

Throughout this book, you'll be invited to answer some questions about yourself, your weight loss goals, your lifestyle, and your eating habits. We've provided space right in this book for your answers. You might prefer to use your own notebook.

Writing down this information provides one of the most important motivational sources you're likely to find during the weeks or months ahead. There's something about putting your thoughts on paper that creates a need, a desire to follow through to successful conclusion.

Moreover, when you commit your thoughts to black and white, you'll be able to read your answers in the future.

So please, don't skip the "Your Turn" sections. And please, *write* your answers, rather than answering them in your head. We'll give you plenty of information to help you change the ending of your weight loss story. But the real change has to come from you. Your desire, your commitment, and your actions are what make the crucial difference.

Decide now to be active, not passive, in your plan to lose weight. Part of this involves looking at yourself honestly. We guarantee you'll use this information faster, more easily and more completely if you make use of the "Your Turn" sections to understand your personal situation better.

Let's get started.

Either here or in your private notebook, answer these questions as candidly and completely as you can:

1. Read over the vignettes about the people at the beginning of this chapter. Pretend that you are the next person whose story appears there. Write the paragraph describing you and your weight issues:

2. Why did you get this book? List your personal reasons.

3. What do you want to accomplish? Be specific.

4. What evidence can you offer that you are really serious about reaching your goals?

2

Here's What Happens
When You Diet

The frightening thought is that dieting may be
the most important cause of obesity!
That would be one hell of a thing to find out.

—**Dean Edell, M.D., medical reporter**

Starving Your Fat and Other Tortures

In 1944, a group of World War II conscientious objectors volunteered for a six-month food deprivation research study. These men were young, bright, and emotionally stable. After two months of eating only half their normal food intake, they had lost half their total body fat—and had become irritable, lethargic, depressed, and preoccupied with food.

As the experiment continued, two men suffered emotional breakdowns. A third, desperate to be released from the program, chopped off the tip of his finger. After the food restrictions ended, the men reported insatiable hunger for months, even when they ate as much as 11,000 calories in one day.

The moral of the experiment to lose weight should be

clear: food deprivation is not the winning solution, even though it appears so perfectly logical: Simply restrict your calorie intake and lose weight.

It works at first. You cheer at each declining pound that fails to appear at your weekly weigh-ins. Before long, though, the weight isn't coming off so quickly. You retaliate and cut your calories further. The fact that you've been carrying the extra weight for ten years doesn't matter. You want to lose it by your birthday, or class reunion, or your mother's visit, regardless of the cost. And so you decide that your fat can't possibly live on cottage cheese and carrot sticks, so you try eating that for a few days.

Then one day you notice a liquid diet in the drugstore. The label says to use it in place of only one or two meals, but surely the weight would come off faster if you substituted this liquid miracle for all three meals. And maybe some of these capsules from the health food store would help. . . .

Thus, you lose weight, maybe a lot, at first. Sure, you're hungry all the time, and yes, you snap at your kids. You have no energy, no interest in anything but your next meal. But that's the price you have to pay for reaching your goals, right?

Wrong. It isn't a price you have to pay. And wrong again—it doesn't help you reach your goals. Let's look closer.

Fat vs. Famine: And The Winner Is . . .

> *My soul is dark with stormy riot,*
> *Directly traceable to diet.*
> **—Samuel Hoffenstein (1890-1947)**

When you reduce your calorie intake drastically, your body doesn't realize you're depriving it intentionally. It reacts as if it's being starved. The body's metabolic rate, the rate at which calories are converted to energy, slows down and conserves fat. This is our bodies' natural way of preserving us during famines and food shortages. But it's the opposite of what anyone on a diet wants!

If your method of dieting is to reduce your calories from "Way-Too-Many" to "Just-What-You-Really-Need," that's fine. But if you diet by reducing calories to less than what your body needs (and therefore deprive yourself of necessary nutrients as well), this book is talking to you.

Avoiding The Low Ebb

How can you tell if your diet is too low in calories? Those food deprivation signals described in the above research study—lethargy, irritability, obsession with the next meal, and constant hunger—are your body's screams for more food. If you don't heed them, your body will say to itself, "I'm in big trouble. I'd better shut down my furnace and conserve these few calories I'm getting just to keep myself alive."

So the more you *deny* yourself needed nutrients, the more your body *fights* by lowering your metabolic rate. It wants to live. That's the bottom line. The body has no way of knowing you're starving it on purpose.

The results can be devastating. You lose muscle as well as fat, and you feel cold, tired and depressed. Your skin and hair get dry. If there aren't enough calories to supply all the body's functions, after all, it chooses to feed the most important. It can't be bothered with keeping you energetic or your hair glossy.

"But wait!" you say. "I always lose weight on very low calorie diets, at least at first. They work!" That depends on your definition of "work." Very low calorie diets can give you an impressive initial weight loss. But what are you losing?

Not fat. You can only lose fat gradually, at about 1/2 to 2 pounds a week. "No way!" you insist. "I lost 7 pounds the first week!"

Ready for some bad news? If your scale shows a pound a day, it's mostly water. *Always.* It might look good on the bathroom scale, but it's meaningless. It's always temporary. You're not losing fat.

Though meaningless in terms of your goals, it's far from a harmless sleight-of-scale. Your body doesn't want that water loss, so it'll start holding on. Diuretics are useless. You'll regain all your water weight and then some. The scale numbers will creep up again.

Of course, if you stay on the very low calorie diet long enough, you'll lose fat—but at what cost? Your body will be weakened with the loss of lean muscle. The risk of gallstones is greater with very low calorie diets, and so is the risk of cardiac arrest.

True, some people need to lose weight quickly because of extreme obesity and individual health risks that outweigh the dangers of very low calorie dieting. Your doctor will advise you if this is true for you.

Even so, the very real danger of heart damage or other medical problems from extremely low calorie diets should make you seek a second or third medical opinion before trying a rapid weight loss program. If you're not at least 30 percent above your ideal weight, please don't consider such a drastic deprivation program.

Here are some more sobering facts:

- Almost half the people who sign up for medically supervised weight loss programs fail to complete them.
- People who lose weight rapidly are three times more likely to gain it back than people who lose weight slowly.
- 90 percent of dieters regain their lost weight within one year.

- 48 million dieters spend $10 billion a year on diet programs and products but have very little visual proof their purchases bought anything other than empty promises and an all-expense paid guilt trip to fat city.
- The single most important factor for keeping lost weight off is *exercise*.

Yo-Yo Dieting

> *It's one of our most human traits in all parts of the world to keep trying the same solution, even when it's not working. You think it's you—not the solution—that's not good enough.*
> **—Margaret Mackenzie, cultural anthropologist**

We've all seen friends go on diet after diet, losing pounds only to gain them back again, often ending up heavier and less healthy than when they started. Maybe we've done this ourselves.

Yo-yo dieting, or "cycling," means losing and regaining weight through repeated start and stop dieting. It's tough on the body and devastating to morale.

If you're a yo-yo dieter, you already know that you regain your weight more quickly each time you lose it. Your body is becoming a real expert at keeping you alive through an onslaught of "famines."

You can't tell this from the scale, but each time you diet you lose more muscle and regain more fat. So your body fat percentage actually increases each time you diet. Even if you return to the same weight, your body is actually fatter!

Your metabolic rate slows with each diet. With years of dieting practice, you might find you're eating very little, and still keeping the pounds on. That's because you've lowered your metabolic rate and (most likely) decreased your lean muscle mass, so you burn calories more slowly than a healthy, non-dieter.

Cellulite: Fancy Fat

Just as gimmicks don't work to get rid of fat, they don't get rid of cellulite, those cottage-cheese-like puckers on the buttocks and the backs of our thighs. That's because—ta da!—cellulite is just fat.

The French word "cellulite" (pronounced "sell-you-leet") was first used in European health spas in the early 1900s. The term came to the United States via a Frenchwoman who owned a beauty salon in New York City. Now we cream, heat and pummel those lumpy bulges with everything from horse-hair mitts and rubberized pants to electrical muscle stimulators and enzyme injections.

Cellulite isn't a medical condition or a cosmetic blemish. There's no structural difference between cellulite and ordinary fat. It looks different because it's right beneath the skin, in fat cell compartments separated by fibrous tissue. When the fat cells increase in size, the fat compartments bulge and get that waffled look. As we age, the outer layers of skin get thinner and less elastic, making the fat cell bulges more apparent.

Sorry, it's not very glamorous. But the good news is that you can take care of it the way you take care of the fat everywhere else on your body—and that's what we'll show you now.

Your Turn: Your Dieting History

On this page or in your private notebook, write honest answers to these questions. Don't let embarrassment stop you from answering fully, because your responses will help you use this book to make permanent changes.

1. Describe the first extreme diet you remember going on. How old were you? How much did you weigh before the diet? How much weight did you lose, and how fast? How much did you weigh a year later?

2. How many times have you gone on extreme diets? How long did you last on each one? Are you lighter or heavier than when you started extreme dieting?

3. How long ago was your most recent extreme diet? Describe what you did or didn't eat, and for how long. How much weight did you lose? How much of that have you regained?

4. How do you feel while you're dieting? Describe your emotions and your physical sensations.

5. Would you like to be free from extreme dieting forever? What eating and exercise changes are you willing to make to accomplish this?

3

Establishing
Realistic Goals

Case Study: Edith

Edith, 49, is 70 pounds above her ideal weight, and a dedicated dieter. The wife of a surgeon, she also has plenty of free time. Though she rarely exercises at home, she frequently enrolls in diet programs and twice a year she enrolls in a weight loss spa. She loses weight, goes home, regains her weight, and does it again.

Far from acting defeated, Edith seems to enjoy her role as self-proclaimed authority when the talk turns to diets, which it inevitably does. She peppers her conversation with cheery references to her latest weight loss feats.

Sitting at breakfast at a weight loss spa after an early morning walk, Edith raved to her walking leader about her favorite diet from last year. "I lost 60 pounds on that diet!" Edith said, chin high with pride.

"Sixty pounds of what?" asked the instructor, who had tried to discuss the difference between pound weight and body fat loss the day before.

"I don't care!" Edith retorted, eyes blazing, chin still high.

Looking Deeper

Clearly, Edith is stuck. She is riding the diet roller coaster. She doesn't even realize how her passion for losing pounds (the more the better), is making her problem worse. Instead of changing her lifestyle, she relies on quick fixes: temporary diets, trips to the spa. Instead of learning about low-fat eating, she pays others to feed her for a time. Instead of making exercise part of her daily life, she uses it short-term to get her weight down.

If, instead, she took to heart the behavior modification programs at the weight loss clinics and took home the recipes and exercise routines from the spas, she wouldn't have to keep repeating her weight loss.

Look at your own patterns of losing and regaining weight. Is there some of Edith in you? Have there been times that the goals you sought were part of the problem, rather than the solution? Did you, like Edith, want to lose "pounds" without caring "pounds of what"?

If so, acknowledge this as part of your past, but let it go. Now's the time to make real changes for your future; you have more information now and you don't have to repeat those diet cycles.

Please don't take the blame for the mind-set that pushed you aboard that unrewarding merry-go-round. If a diet fails, society tells you it's your fault, that you didn't try hard enough. But now you see the truth: 90 percent of temporary, restrictive diets fail because they don't teach you to make permanent changes in your eating behavior and energy expenditure levels.

No wonder dieters are confused. Cultural role models project conflicting goals and impossible images. Magazines promote the latest quick weight loss diet, side by side with recipes for double fudge chocolate cake. Anorexic fashion models parade in clothing that a woman with hips, thighs and bosom could never wear. Size six aerobics instructors bemoan a gained pound. Celebrities reshape their breasts and bottoms as well as their noses. Our culture hates fat with a disgust that is difficult to understand—especially since 30 percent of us are overweight by society's standards.

There's No Body Like Your Body

So you're not Jane Fonda, Sylvester Stallone or Cher. Chances are, you never were. Humans come in many varieties of body types and sizes. Stop driving yourself crazy by wishing you could trade bodies with someone else. Instead, work to make your body the best, healthiest and fittest it can be. Once you've adopted a low-fat eating pattern and a balanced fitness exercise program, you're making powerful changes. Lighten up your attitude about how much you weigh or how fast you lose.

How Much Can You Reshape Your Body?

Though we come in infinite variations, our bodies fall reasonably well into three basic body types:

An ectomorph has a tendency to stay thin whatever (almost) her eating habits. A mesomorph is compact and puts on muscle easily. An endomorph has difficulty losing weight even with exercise and healthy eating.

Our culture reveres the ectomorph. A long-legged, slender ballet dancer or a fashion model is a good example of the ectomorph body type. But be aware that many of these people have starved themselves into the ectomorphic look and aren't there by nature.

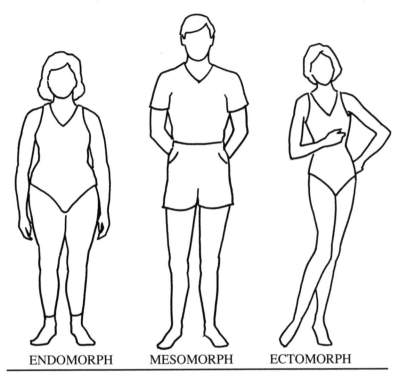

ENDOMORPH   MESOMORPH   ECTOMORPH

Look around you and count ectomorphs. How many do you see on the street or in the shopping mall? Right. Very few. They're a small percentage of the population, and perhaps that's why we idealize them so. But if your body shape—inherited from your parents—has large thighs and short legs, no amount of dieting or exercise will transform you into Cher.

Where you carry your fat stores is also genetic. If your parents have large bellies, chances are you carry your fat there, also. If they have thick waists, you'll just frustrate yourself trying to be Scarlett O'Hara. You can reshape your body within your genetic limits through low-fat eating and exercise, but you can't change those genetic limits any more than you can change your height or the length of your fingers.

Does that mean you throw this book in the trash and go

back to chocolate-covered marshmallows? No. It means you look at yourself, your parents, and your grandparents. Look at the bone structure and body type you've inherited. Then you set your personal role model as the best body that your body can be.

Realize that an active, fit lifestyle is your most powerful magic wand for creating the best body you can have. Don't resign yourself to Grandma's large hips if she spends the day eating. Tell yourself, "My body will look just like Grandma's if I lead a sedentary life and overeat. Now let's see what it can look like if I exercise wisely, consistently and eat right." (And for Grandma's health and because you love her, how about sharing this book with her and making a date to go walking together?)

The Myth Of "Ideal" Weights

Gretchen, 50, is an avid swimmer and cyclist. She also lifts weights to strengthen her legs and upper body. She is proud of her strong, sturdy, youthful appearance. At 5'8", she weighs 160 pounds, and her body fat is a healthy 21 percent. Yet she was startled to read on a "desirable weight" chart that she is considered overweight for her frame. She rushed to her doctor. Should she lose weight?

Have you ever wanted to rip the Metropolitan Life Insurance Company's height and weight table to shreds? That's the chart that says if you're x feet y inches tall, you'd better not weigh more than z pounds.

Go ahead, rip up the charts. For the same reasons that the scale doesn't do the job in telling you if you're losing fat, the height and weight table is inadequate for telling you if you're at a healthy weight.

Why? It gives you a range of pounds. Pounds of what? The chart doesn't differentiate between fat and muscle weight.

1959 Metropolitan Height & Weight Tables

MEN

Height Feet Inches		Small Frame	Medium Frame	Large Frame
5	1	105-113	111-122	119-134
5	2	108-116	114-126	122-137
5	3	111-119	117-129	125-141
5	4	114-122	120-132	128-146
5	5	117-126	123-136	131-149
5	6	121-130	127-140	135-154
5	7	125-134	131-146	140-159
5	8	129-138	135-149	144-163
5	9	133-143	139-153	148-167
5	10	137-147	143-158	152-172
5	11	141-151	147-163	157-177
6	0	145-155	151-168	161-182
6	1	149-160	155-173	166-187
6	2	153-164	160-178	171-192
6	3	157-168	165-183	175-197

WOMEN

Height Feet Inches		Small Frame	Medium Frame	Large Frame
4	9	90-97	94-106	102-118
4	10	92-100	97-109	105-121
4	11	95-103	100-112	108-124
5	0	98-106	103-115	111-127
5	1	101-109	106-118	114-130
5	2	104-112	109-122	117-134
5	3	107-115	112-126	121-138
5	4	110-119	116-131	125-142
5	5	114-123	120-135	129-146
5	6	118-127	124-139	133-150
5	7	122-131	128-143	137-154
5	8	126-136	132-147	141-159
5	9	130-140	136-151	145-164
5	10	134-144	140-155	149-169

Nude weights

Reprinted courtesy of Metropolitan Life Insurance Company

1983 Metropolitan Height & Weight Tables

MEN

Height Feet Inches		Small Frame	Medium Frame	Large Frame
5	1	123-129	126-136	133-145
5	2	125-131	128-138	135-148
5	3	130-136	133-143	140-153
5	4	132-138	135-145	142-156
5	5	134-140	137-148	144-160
5	6	136-142	139-151	146-164
5	7	138-145	142-154	149-168
5	8	140-148	145-157	152-172
5	9	142-151	148-160	155-176
5	10	144-154	151-163	158-180
5	11	146-157	154-166	161-184
6	0	149-160	157-170	164-188
6	1	152-164	160-174	168-192
6	2	155-168	164-178	172-197
6	3	158-172	167-182	176-202

WOMEN

4	9	99-108	106-118	115-128
4	10	100-110	108-120	117-131
4	11	101-112	110-123	119-134
5	0	103-115	112-126	122-137
5	1	105-118	115-129	125-140
5	2	108-121	118-132	128-144
5	3	111-124	121-135	131-148
5	4	114-127	124-138	134-152
5	5	117-130	127-141	137-156
5	6	120-133	130-144	140-160
5	7	123-136	133-147	143-164
5	8	126-139	136-150	146-167
5	9	129-142	139-153	149-170
5	10	132-145	142-156	152-173

Nude weights

Reprinted courtesy of Metropolitan Life Insurance Company

A body builder would weigh in as obese according to the chart, though he might have only 6 percent body fat.   A chronic dieter who is light in weight but has lost much of her lean muscle mass would be classified as normal, although her body fat might be 35 percent.

Doctors regularly use the height/weight tables even though they provide little information about health. Rather, they are longevity tables: they predict *mortality.* And though the tables have data on millions of people, these are only people who buy life insurance. Moreover, only a paltry 12 percent of the sample are women.

As you can see from comparing the 1959 and 1983 versions of the Metropolitan Life table, carrying a few more pounds is considered healthier now than it was a few decades ago. Why? Metropolitan Life discovered that people who were underweight had a higher death rate that those who were a few pounds overweight.

It's likely that the increased death rate among thin people was caused by cigarette smoking or undiagnosed diseases, such as cancer—not from too few pounds. But likewise, does having a few extra pounds mean an earlier death, or are there other factors we need to examine?

In fact, studies are finding that *where* people carry their fat has a more significant impact on health than how much of it they have. People who carry fat in their upper bodies—the male pattern—seem to have more health risk problems, such as diabetes and high blood pressure. People who carry fat in their lower bodies—the female pattern—appear to have less health risk. Upper body fat is also easier to lose than lower body fat.

So instead of clinging to the ideal weight charts, follow a healthy lifestyle and reduce your body fat. The body that results, whether or not it matches the height/weight charts or our cultural ideal, is indeed "ideal" for you.

Setpoint Theory

"Setpoint" is one of the new and perhaps brightest new theories which sheds new light on why we become over-weight, and how we can best lose weight.

Setpoint has been variously described by medical re-searchers as a point, perhaps a *range* might be more accurate, at which each individual's weight will tend to return when not dieting or overeating.

If true, the setpoint theory could explain why most people who don't worry about their weight don't vary much month to month, even though they don't count calories. It also might reveal why ectomorphs stay thin and endomorphs stabilize at a higher weight, even when they don't overeat.

Finding Your Ideal Weight

To determine your setpoint, look at what you usually weigh when you're not dieting, overeating, or coping with a personal crisis. That's probably the midpoint of your range. Now consider what you weighed when you were eating the most and exercising the least: the high end.

During adulthood:

I have rarely weighed less than   _____
I have rarely weighed more than   _____
My setpoint is likely to be   _____

To find the low end, don't look at the lowest temporary weight you ever attained. If you couldn't maintain that weight, it's lower than your setpoint and bound to cause frustration if you try to achieve it again. Instead, look at what you weighed during your time of best eating and exercise habits. That's probably the lower end of your setpoint range, and it's a realistic goal you can reach by changing your food choices and activity level.

Can You Reset Your Setpoint?

Since setpoint itself is just a theory, the answer to whether you can *reset* your setpoint is equally theoretical. Yet, the research seems promising. Exercise appears to lower setpoint, dieting does not.

There is an abundance of evidence that you can lower your weight*within* your setpoint range by permanently changing your metabolic rate through regular, frequent aerobic exercise and strength training.

If healthful eating and exercise habits have not been a part of your life so far, you might not know the low end of your setpoint range or even what to aim for. That's all right—you're on your way to making this discovery. Until then, avoid setting unrealistic goals that don't take your personal body type, shape, and setpoint range into account. Make friends with your body, and embark on the journey towards your personal best.

4

Less Fat In You,
Less Fat On You

The food you eat today is walking and talking tomorrow.

—Jack La Lanne, fitness celebrity

Why A Calorie Is Not A Calorie

Rosie and Denise, both 34, decided to reduce their calories safely and moderately to 1500 calories a day. Rosie was careful to eat less than 500 calories of fat, or 30 percent of her total. Most of the calories in her eating program came from complex carbohydrates. Denise stuck to a 1,500-calorie diet, but ate more fatty foods like hamburgers and luncheon meats. Both took the same aerobics classes. At the end of six weeks, Rosie had lost seven pounds, Denise had lost two.

Walter, 43, had been eating about 40 percent of his calories as fat. He decreased that percentage to 25 percent fat by changing the type of food he ate, but not the amount. After three months, he had lost six pounds without reducing his total calorie intake.

We used to think that 3,500 calories equal one pound of

body weight. We used to believe that if you eat 3,500 calories more than you need, you'll gain a pound. If you eat 3,500 calories less than you need, you'll lose a pound.

Researchers now believe the assumption that calories are calories, whatever their source, is faulty. Recent studies are beginning to show that the fat we eat is more likely than other food components to turn into body fat. Dietary fat is easily stored. Reducing the amount of fat you eat, then, is more important than reducing your total food intake.

What's more, by reducing your fat intake, you'll trim from your lifestyle what the surgeon general has claimed is the "leading cause of disease."

In a scathing 1988 report, the surgeon general went on to say that fat should be reduced in most people's diets by choosing foods relatively low in fats.

So now you've got a double-barreled reason to reduce fat. Let that sink in: *Less fat. If you want to lose body fat, put less fat in your mouth.*

How Fat Turns To Fat

The trip from mouth to fat cells is fast and simple. That's because the fat in your food is more easily and quickly converted to body fat than is protein or carbohydrate. Fat on your lips easily becomes fat on your hips.

Want some proof? In one study, groups of men were intentionally overfed large quantities of food. The men who ate large, high-carbohydrate meals gained 30 pounds in seven months. The men who ate large, high-fat meals gained 30 pounds in three months. The high-fat eaters even had fewer total calories! Clearly, how much fat you eat, more than the total calories, determines how much fat you wear.

Gram for gram, fat also contains more than twice the calories of protein or carbohydrates. Chances are, if your eating pattern is high in fat, it's also high in calories. That's a double whammy!

On the lighter side (so to speak), if you eat meals low in fat and high in complex carbohydrates, you can eat more and still lose. You won't go hungry on a low-fat diet.

Fat Countdown

Most Americans eat 40 percent or more of their calories as fat. We'd be healthier and trimmer if we reduced that to 30 percent or below. Aim for 20 percent, and you'll have an easier time staying under 30 percent, even if you have an occasional slip.

Here's a helpful tip: try to buy foods that are less than 30 percent fat. Then, putting together low-fat meals requires very little planning. Sure, you'll want the occasional avocado, chunk of cheese, or spoonful of peanut butter. But aim mostly for items under 30 percent fat. The more aware you are of the fat content of your foods, the more successful you'll be at making small changes in your eating patterns.

How Much Fat Is In Your Foods?

How much fat is in your foods? Look at the following chart of foods Americans typically eat. The numbers will boggle. For a more detailed fat gram counter, check the diet section of your local bookstore or health food store. Get used to counting fat grams, not calories.

Cutting Down Obvious Fat

One easy way to start is to trim the visible fat from food and cut down on high-fat foods, such as: butter, oil, whole-milk dairy products, fatty cuts of meat, luncheon meats, poultry skin, egg yolks, salad dressings, cream sauces, nuts, chips, olives and avocadoes.

FAT CONTENT OF VARIOUS FOODS

FOOD	AMOUNT	TOTAL FAT IN GRAMS	TOTAL FAT IN TEASPOONS*
VEGETABLES		none	none
FRUITS		none	none
except:			
Olives	5 small	4	1
Avocado	½	16	3
GRAIN PRODUCTS			
Pasta (no egg)	1 c. cooked	0.5	—
Rice			
white	1 c. cooked	0.2	—
brown	1 c. cooked	0.9	—
Breads, average	1 slice	0.6	—
French, Italian	1 slice	0.6	—
Cornbread	1 piece	3.8	¾
White	1 slice	0.7	—
Whole wheat	1 slice	0.7	—
Raisin	1 slice	0.6	—
Rye, pumpernickel	1 slice	0.3	—
Hamburger roll	1	2.2	½
Granola	½ c. commercial	8	1½
NUTS & SEEDS			
Cashews	1 oz. = 14 large	13.1	2½
Walnuts	1 oz. = 15 halves	15.1	3
Pistachio	1 oz. = 50	16.1	3¼
Almonds	1 oz. = 25	16.2	3¼
Sunflower seeds	¼ c.	16.8	3¼
Peanuts (dry-roasted)	¼ c.	17.6	3½
Filberts	1 oz. = 25	19.1	3¾
Pecans	1 oz. = 24 halves	22	4½
Macadamia nuts	1 oz. = 12	23.5	4¾

*rounded values

FOOD	AMOUNT	TOTAL FAT IN GRAMS	TOTAL FAT IN TEASPOONS
LEGUMES	1 c.	less than 1	—
MILK PRODUCTS			
Skim milk, buttermilk	1 c.	0.4	—
Frozen yogurt	½ c.	1.5	¼
Sherbet	½ c	1.9	¼
1% milk	1 c.	2.6	½
Ice milk	½ c.	2.8	½
2% milk	1 c.	5	1
Low fat yogurt	1 c.	4	1
Regular yogurt	1 c.	8	1½
Ice cream, regular	½ c.	8	1½
Whole milk	1 c.	9	1¾
Ice cream, rich	½ c.	15	3
Half & half	½ c.	16	3
Sour cream	½ c.	16	3
Whipping cream	½ c.	24	5
CHEESES			
Cottage cheese, 2%	½ c.	2.2	½
Reduced Calorie Laughing Cow	1 oz.	3	½
Mozzarella, skim	1 oz.	2	½
Lite-Line (Borden)	1 oz.	3	½
Hickory Lite-Line	1 oz.	3	½
Weight-Watcher	1 oz.	2	½
Ricotta, part skim	1 oz.	2	½
Cottage cheese, 4%	½ c.	4.2	1
Mozzarella, part skim	1 oz.	4.5	1
Light cream cheese	1 oz.	5	1
Parmesan (grated)	¼ c.	6	1¼
Mozzarella	1 oz.	6	1¼
Feta	1 oz.	6	1¼
Green River cheddar	1 oz.	7	1½
Neufchatel cream cheese	1 oz.	7	1½
Ricotta	1 oz.	4	1

FOOD	AMOUNT	TOTAL FAT IN GRAMS	TOTAL FAT IN TEASPOONS
CHEESES, continued			
Cheddar, gruyere, jack, blue, etc.	1 oz.	9-10	2
Cream cheese	1 oz.	10	2
Brie, Camembert	1 oz.	13-15	3
FISH & SHELLFISH, POULTRY, MEATS (COOKED)			
White flesh fish (cod, halibut, sole, snapper, perch, haddock, trout)	3 oz.	0-1	—
Shellfish	3 oz.	0-1	—
Tuna, packed in water	3 oz.	1	¼
Salmon, pink	3 oz.	3.2	¾
Chicken, turkey, no skin, white	3 oz.	4	1
Veal, venison	3 oz.	5	1
Tuna, canned in oil	3 oz.	8	1½
Bacon	2 strips	7.5	1½
Chicken, turkey, no skin, dark	3 oz.	8.4	1¾
Beef, flank, round, sirloin, 10% fat	3 oz.	8.5	1¾
Spareribs	3 small	10	2
Salmon, chinook	3 oz.	13.3	2⅔
Pork, lamb	3 oz.	12	2½
Ground beef, 25% fat	3 oz.	21.5	4½
LUNCHEON MEATS			
Turkey products	1 oz.	1.5	¼
Bologna	1 oz.	8	1½
Salami, dry	1 oz.	10	2
Wiener	one	13	2½
EGGS			
White	1	0.5	—
Yolk	1	5.5	1
Whole egg	1	6	1¼

FOOD	AMOUNT	TOTAL FAT IN GRAMS	TOTAL FAT IN TEASPOONS
FATS & SPREADS			
Catsup, mustard	1 Tbsp.	less than 1	—
Imitation mayonnaise	1 Tbsp.	5	1
Diet margarine	1 Tbsp.	5	1
Miracle Whip	1 Tbsp.	6.9	1¼
Soft margarine, whipped	1 Tbsp.	8	1½
Peanut butter	1 Tbsp.	8	1½
Mayonnaise	1 Tbsp.	11	2
Margarine	1 Tbsp.	12	2½
Butter	1 Tbsp.	14	3
Oils—all	1 Tbsp.	14	3
SALAD DRESSINGS			
Commercial "low-calorie," "diet"	1 Tbsp.	1	¼
French	1 Tbsp.	5.4	1
Roquefort, 1000 island	1 Tbsp.	7.6	1½
Italian	1 Tbsp.	8.4	1¾
SNACKS			
Bagel	1	less than 1	—
Popcorn, plain	1 c.	0.3	—
Pretzels	10	less than 1	—
Melba toast, matzoh	1	less than 1	—
Muffin, whole wheat	1	1.1	¼
Saltines	4	1.4	¼
Gingersnaps	4	1.2	¼
Corn chips	½ c.	6	1¼
Popcorn, buttered	1 c.	2	½
Triscuits	4	3	½
Chocolate chip cookies	2	4.4	1
Oreo cookies	2	4.5	1
Chocolate cupcake	1	5	1
Doughnut, raised	1	9.9	2
Peach crisp	1 slice	6.4	1¼

FOOD	AMOUNT	TOTAL FAT IN GRAMS	TOTAL FAT IN TEASPOONS
SNACKS, continued			
Chocolate bar	1 oz.	10	2
Croissant, plain	1	10	2
Double crust peach pie	1 slice	12	2¼
Potato chips	1 oz.	12.5	2½
FAST FOODS			
Pizza, cheese, mushroom	1 slice	4.4	1
Typical milkshake, chocolate	1	8.4	1¾
Typical hamburger	1	10	2
Typical cheeseburger	1	14	3
French fries	1 serving	14	3
Big Mac hamburger	1	33	6½

Fast Food Facts by Marion Franz, R.D., M.S., Copyright © 1990, International Diabetes Center with permission of its publisher, DCI Publishing.

You also want to modify your cooking style to keep from adding fat. Anytime you add oil, as in deep frying or sauteing, you're doubling—sometimes tripling—the calories of your ingredients. And all those extra calories are fat.

Instead, lightly oil your pan with the end of a stick of butter or margarine, or a pastry brush dipped in oil. Try non-stick cookware and skip the fat altogether. Or cook in broth or tomato juice. Your microwave oven is a terrific aid for fat-free cooking.

You can remove more fat from soups and stews if you prepare them several hours early and refrigerate them. The fat will harden on the surface, and you can easily remove it before reheating. If you don't have that much time, at least let the food cool and skim the fat.

Choose a milk or yogurt that's lower in fat than what you

ordinarily buy. Ideally, use non-fat, but if you're used to high-fat, make the change in smaller steps.

For example, if you're used to cream in your coffee or cereal, try whole milk for a few weeks and then switch to low-fat. Once you lose the taste for the higher fat product—and you will—you'll be able to make the transition to healthier non-fat more easily.

Reading Labels

A frustration you'll face is recognizing fats that aren't visible. How can you know that a croissant has 12 times as much fat and 50 percent more calories than an English muffin of the same weight? How can you tell if the luncheon meat that screams "LITE!" from its colorful label is really a low-fat alternative? How do you decide if you should take a chance on that frozen pizza?

Food labeling laws are far from perfect, but you can figure out the percentage of fat in any food item that provides you with the fat grams and the total calories per serving. Here's how you can do it:

1. Multiply the grams of fat listed on the label by nine(the number of calories in each gram of fat). The result is the total number of calories from fat per serving.
2. Divide that number by the total calories per serving, also listed on the label. This gives you the percent of calories from fat.

For example, one brand of oat bran muffin mix has five grams of fat per serving. The total fat calories per serving, then, is 5 x 9 = 45. The total calories per serving = 140; 45

divided by 140 = .32. So this brand of muffin is 32 percent fat—and that's before you butter it. That's not awful, but not "low-fat," either.

However, compare that muffin to a Great Start Sausage, Egg, and Cheese on a Biscuit frozen breakfast product with 470 calories and 29 grams fat. Come on, figure it out: 29 x 9 equals ? Right! 261. Now divide your result by 470. What did you get? That's right, a whopping 56% fat. They call that a "great start" to the day? Indeed.

Go ahead, take a notepad and a pocket calculator to the supermarket. Make a game of it: Can you find the highest and lowest fat products in a food category you use frequently? We guarantee surprises!

If you'd rather not fiddle with a calculator, here's a simple shortcut: look for foods with less than three grams of fat for every 100 calories. That gives you a safe 27 percent fat maximum.

Read The Fine Print

Test: If a luncheon meat label states "80 percent fat free" or better, it's a healthful addition to a low-fat diet, right? Be careful! Don't take low-fat label claims at face value without doing the fat percentage test for yourself.

"What!" you exclaim, after doing the fat test, "77 percent of its calories come from fat! How can they lie like that?"

Shame on those food companies for misleading us, but they're not lying. They're measuring fat content by weight—a useless measure—instead of by percentage of total calories, the measurement you want.

When you look at the calories from fat, you get the bad news: that "80% fat free" turkey bologna is 77 percent fat by calories. One brand of chicken bologna greases you with 90 percent of its calories from fat! Since you're trying to reduce your fat intake to less than 30 percent of your total calories, you won't find any health bargains here.

Don't count on the words "lite" or "lean" to help you out. The fat may have been reduced by 25 percent, but that leaves plenty to swallow. Some brands with "lite," "lean" or "light & lean" in their names have up to 15 grams of fat in two slices.

Luncheon meats are one of the worst offenders. After all, if they told the honest truth, what fat-conscious shopper would buy them? But they're not the only offenders. Zap some of the so-called "light" frozen entrées with your calculator.

Budget Gourmet Light entrées, for example, all say "95 % Fat Free," and in smaller print, "contains 5% fat." Sounds good. Now get out your magnifying glass and read the nutrition disclosure. The lasagna, you'll find, is 300 calories and 13 grams fat. $13 \times 9 = 117$, divided by $300 = 39$ percent fat!

How can they claim "5% fat"? Again, they're advertising the amount of fat by weight, not calories. Those 117 calories only weigh 5 percent of the total entree. Big deal, right?

Vote with your wallet against companies that attempt to disarm your ability to make sound, nutritional choices by providing misleading information. If you can't give up luncheon meats, look for those with only one or two grams of fat per two-ounce serving.

Fake Fat: Bogus Or Bonanza?

Food chemists have burned the midnight oil creating fake fat so that we can give up our fat and eat it, too. This fake fat tastes like fat, but isn't fat. One fat substitute is made from egg whites and milk and lets us eat lower-calorie frozen desserts without guilt. Is this the ice cream fanatic's salvation?

Doubtful. The benefits we'll get from fake fat are just the tip of the ice cream. Much of our fat intake comes from cooked fats, and this fat substitute is not heat-stable, and therefore it cannot be used in cooked products.

More important, eating fake fat does nothing to cut down your craving for high-fat foods. Look at fake sugar: we've had artificial sweeteners for 80 years, and we're fatter and more sweets-addicted than ever. Surely you've seen folks eating a second slice of cheesecake while stirring artificial sweetener into their coffee. Likewise, don't expect fake fat to accomplish much more than making us complacent about the amount of real fat we're eating.

It might not be the easy way out, but it's the only way out: reduce the amount of fat you eat. You'll get used to the taste of lower-fat foods. Honest. You may even prefer them! You'll certainly like the changes in your body when you cut down your fat—in you and on you.

Tips for Reducing Your Dietary Fat

Here are some easy ways to reduce the fat in your diet:

• **Buy a hot air popcorn popper**, and don't add butter later. A cup of plain popcorn has only 25 calories, is high-fiber and filling, and tastes great even without butter, especially when it's fresh and hot.

• **Traveling by plane?** If you phone your airline ahead, they'll substitute a low-fat meal for the food your fellow passengers will be eating. (And you might get a better meal!)

• **Substitute sour cream** with non-fat cottage cheese and yogurt, whipped in the blender and seasoned with chives, herbs, onion or garlic.

• **Top your pancakes** with warmed applesauce or banana slices instead of butter and syrup.

• **Warm your bread in the microwave**, and it'll be moist even without butter.

• **Steam or microwave** vegetables instead of sauteing.

• **Dress salads with rice vinegar** (available in the Oriental food section of your supermarket), a tasty seasoning even without oil.

• **Use egg whites** instead of whole eggs in recipes.

• **Top baked potatoes or pasta** with non-fat yogurt or chopped, cooked vegetables, or both. Or lemon juice with chopped onion.

• **Substitute non-fat milk** for cream in soup, and puree a portion of the vegetables to thicken the soup.

• **Grate and sprinkle cheese over casseroles**, pasta and sandwiches—wherever you usually add cheese slices or chunks. You'll get the flavor with less fat and fewer calories.

• **Mix cooked brown rice or diced vegetables** with the chopped meat in meat loaf or hamburger to increase carbohydrates and reduce fat and calories.

• **Take a low-fat cooking class.** You'll be surprised by the variety of tasty recipes.

• **Double the size** of a time-consuming low-fat recipe and freeze the left over food for a future meal.

Your Turn: Your Low-Fat Resolutions

Here or in your private notebook, answer these questions to help you lower your consumption of dietary fat.

1. List favorite high-fat foods you're not willing to give up.

2. List high-fat foods that you are willing to give up.

3. List several high-fat foods that you are willing to eat less often or in smaller amounts.

4. How can you change your cooking style to reduce your fat intake? Be specific.

5. Assemble a few prepared foods that you eat regularly. Figure out the percentage of calories from fat in each item. List the results here. Put a slash mark through any items you're ready to give up due to excess fat.

6. Look over the tips on how to reduce fat. Which ones can you put into action this week?

7. What else are you willing to do to bring your fat intake to under 30 percent?

5

Taking Measure
Of
The Enemy

Ed, 48, joined a health club three months ago, and has been working out daily since then. He alternates weight training with aerobics classes, and uses a NordicTrack cross-country ski exerciser when he can't get to the club. "I didn't lose a pound until last week—but my body shape has changed completely! My chest is bigger, my abdomen is flatter, my butt is higher."

Judy and Susan each weigh 130 pounds at 5'4". Yet Judy's dress size is two sizes smaller than Susan's, and no one would guess they weigh the same. Judy walks four miles almost every day, and strength-trains alternate evenings. Susan watches television.

Scale Savvy

The scale may not be your best ally in your efforts to slim down. Perhaps you saw it as a foe in the past, as you stood on one foot trying to make the numbers go lower. And you were tempted to throw it down the stairs or put it in the cat box when it stubbornly refused to acknowledge how "good" you'd been on your diet. The scale measures weight, so it tells you how much progress you're making, right?

Not always.

This book could have been titled, *The Only Fat Loss Book You'll Ever Need*, but would you have picked it up then? "I'm not fat, just a little overweight," you say in a huff. The point is, whether you think you have 5 pounds or 50 or 150 to lose, you want to lose body fat.

When you step on the scale, it doesn't tell you what you want to know: "How much body fat did I lose (or gain)?" The scale weighs your bones, muscles, and organs. It weighs your blood, the water in your cells, the food you're digesting. Oh yes, it also weighs your body fat. But if the scale says you weigh two pounds less (or more) one morning, how do you know if those two pounds are water weight, muscle change, body fat, or day-to-day fluctuation? You don't.

How Fat Am I?

More important than your scale weight is your body composition, which means the proportion of lean versus fat. This is given in the form of a body fat percentage, as the table on the next page shows.

Hydrostatic Testing

You can get your body fat tested at a health club or sports medicine facility in one of several ways. Hydrostatic (underwater) weighing is complicated, but the most accurate.

The procedure involves a rather simple concept of water displacement first described by Greek mathematician and inventor, Archimedes, who discovered the principle of displacement. Without getting technical, the water displacement method is based on the fact that densities of bone and muscle tissue are higher than water while fat is less dense that water. Therefore, a person with more bone and muscle mass will weigh more in water and thus have a higher bone density and lower percent of body fat.

The testing procedure is simple: you're weighed on land and you're weighed again while submerged in water. Using a standard formula, the amount of your body fat can quickly be determined. In fact, by the time you've climbed out of the water and toweled off, you have your body fat percentage. If the idea of being underwater for a few seconds frightens you, though, you're less likely to get an accurate reading because you will resist exhaling all your air. A good tester will be reassuring as well as competent.

PERCENT BODY FAT CLASSIFICATIONS		
CLASSIFICATION	MALE	FEMALE
Lean	<8%	<13%
Optimal	8-15%	13-20%
Slightly overfat	16-20%	21-25%
Fat	21-24%	26-32%
Obese (overfat)	≥25%	≥32%
Long distance runners	4-9%	6-15%
Wrestlers	4-10%	—
Gymnasts	4-10%	10-17%
Body builders (elite)	6-10%	10-17%
Swimmers	5-11%	14-24%
Basketball athletes	7-11%	18-27%
Canoers/kayakers	11-15%	18-24%
Tennis players	14-17%	19-22%

Reprinted from *Fitness and Sports Medicine—An Introduction*, 1990, © Bull Publishing Company. Sources: Adapted from: Lohman TG. The Use of Skinfold to Estimate Body Fatness on Children and Youth. JOPERD November-December, 1987, pp. 98-102; Fleck SJ. Body Composition of Elite American Athletes. Am J Sports Med 11:398, 1983; Wilmore JH. The Physiology Basis of the Conditioning Process. Boston: Allyn and Bacon, Inc., 1982.

Skin Fold Measurement

Simpler, but slightly less accurate, is skin fold measurement. This test is performed with calipers, an instrument with a pair of movable, curved legs used to measure the diameter or thickness.

The tester holds a section of skin fold from several different sites, such as the hip and the back of the arm, and measures the subcutaneous (under the skin) fat.

The accuracy of this method is open to criticism because it depends more on the skill of the person performing the test rather than the instrument itself.

Still, watching those measurements get smaller and smaller can provide you with a useful record and an important source of weight loss motivation.

Electrical Impedance

Another method is electrical impedance. The tester sends a small electrical current through your body—you don't feel a thing—and measures the body's resistance to that current. The higher the resistance, the more body fat, because electricity travels more easily through lean tissue than fat. The accuracy here is similar to skin fold measurement with an experienced tester.

As people get more concerned with knowing their body fat percentages, both simpler and more sophisticated tests will be developed. Meanwhile, the easiest tool for measuring whether you're losing body fat is a tape measure. The second easiest way is to judge the fit of your clothes. Both are more accurate than the scale.

Help! I'm Gaining Weight!

Felicia, 22, bicycles to her college classes 10 miles from home, does martial arts twice a week, and hikes with a backpack on weekends. In high school, her weight was within average range, but her main physical activity was opening the refrigerator door. The jeans that fit her snugly before are now too large. All her friends comment on how she has slimmed down. Yet the scale says she weighs five pounds more.

The scale's message is not just inadequate, it might be downright deceptive. Some people, like Felicia, actually find that they gain weight when they start developing strength and muscle mass. Yet they appear slimmer and firmer, and friends remark about how lean and fit they look. They are actually losing inches and body fat and gaining muscle weight.

This is because muscle weighs more than fat. You can test this yourself the next time you cut up a chicken for dinner. Remove all the fat and put it in a glass of water. It's so light it floats. But yuk, that's the part you don't want on your hips. Now look at the chicken thigh—dense, muscular, and so heavy it would sink right to the bottom of that glass of water. Likewise, the fat you wear on your body is lighter in weight than your heavier muscle tissue, but it looks soft and puffy.

As you lose fat and gain muscle through your aerobic and strength training program, your scale might not show the difference at first—but your tape measure will. Like Ed and Felicia, you'll find your body is reshaping itself with lean muscle. You'll pull your belt in a notch or two, even though the scale has no comment.

Don't bury your head in the scales! Rethink your attitude. Work to change your fat/lean proportions instead of simply dropping pounds. Keep your body lean by avoiding crash dieting. Try to lose only one or two pounds a week. Exercise to burn fat and gain muscle.

6

Choosing An Eating Plan That Fits Your Lifestyle

Nothing can help. There are no substitutes.
Sometimes I say there are so I can live.
But I know better. Only food can feed;
Not air, not dust, not water through a sieve.

—Abbie Huston Evans, poet (1881-1983)

Eating For Life

We're not asking you to give up food. We're not even asking you to go on a diet, because a diet implies that sooner or later, you'll go off the diet. And you'll have less than 1 in 20 chance of keeping the lost pounds off.

Our society diets constantly, and we get fatter and fatter, not thinner and thinner. So a word of honest advice: Let go of the word "diet" from your solution to being overweight. Instead, substitute the idea of a lifelong balanced eating plan.

Weight loss success doesn't depend on finding the right temporary eating restriction; it depends on finding a well-balanced eating plan that fits into your lifestyle, and incorporates regular strength and aerobic exercise into your daily life.

Freeing yourself from yo-yo dieting and learning how to eat for life is essential to winning the battle of the bulges. Look at your present food habits as companions—let's call them "roommates"—in an eating lifestyle you chose some time ago. Maybe you enjoy them and like having them with you. Maybe they're comfortable and habitual, especially in times of stress or loneliness. Maybe you're indifferent to these roommates. Perhaps it's too much trouble to replace them. Or you hate these roommates, but you feel stuck.

Just remember, they're only roommates. You chose them before you knew the life you really wanted, and you didn't marry them or give birth to them, thank goodness. If some of them don't fit your new goals and lifestyle, you can decide to part company. Let's take a closer look at how this diet plan relates to you personally.

Your Turn: Diagnosing Your Eating Lifestyle

On this page or in your private notebook, list your typical meals and snacks for four days. If you can't do this from memory, take the next four days to record what you eat. Include approximate amounts of food you eat.

Don't try to change your eating habits to make them look better on the page! Just record your normal eating pattern. The first step towards making a change is honestly appraising what it is that needs to be changed. As you fill out this four-day log sheet, answer the following questions:

1. Which of the foods that you eat regularly do you really love?

2. Which are just convenience foods?

3. Which are comfort foods in times of stress or loneliness?

4. Which are habitual foods you don't really care about?

5. Which foods do you over-indulge in?

6. At what time(s) of day do you tend to over-indulge or eat foods you regret later?

7. Which foods seem to set up a craving for more, instead of satisfying you?

8. If you could make just one major change in your eating habits, what would it be? Be specific.

9. What smaller changes could you start making right away?

Four Day Eating Diary

Day 1

Breakfast

Lunch

Dinner

Snacks

Four Day Eating Diary
Day 2

Breakfast

Lunch

Dinner

Snacks

Four Day Eating Diary
Day 3

Breakfast

Lunch

Dinner

Snacks

Four Day Eating Diary

Day 4

Breakfast

Lunch

Dinner

Snacks

Choosing A Lifelong Eating Plan

It's nitty gritty time. We've told you what doesn't work for lifelong weight control. Now let's look at what does work. Here are the components of a lifelong eating plan that is nourishing, keeps your body low in fat, and keeps your energy levels high.

Start With The Basics: Good Nutrition

The more "nutrient-dense" your food choices, the better. That means you get more bang for the buck, or, more accurately, more nutrition for the calories. Seek foods that give you the greatest rate of return on your calorie investment.

The closer foods are to their natural, unprocessed state, the more nutrients they have. That doesn't mean we have to shop in health food stores or buy straight from the farm. Simply choose fresh vegetables over canned, whole grains over refined, and "scratch" recipes over prepared foods.

Avoid burying foods in fats, sugars and sauces that add calories. Choose bananas rather than banana cream pie. Drink milk rather than milk shakes. Eat baked potato without sour cream. Enjoy vegetables without cheese sauce.

We also want a variety and balance of nutrients. You can find several good, easy-to-read nutrition books in our bibliography at the end of this book.

But for now, here's the easiest, quickest way to help guarantee nutritional balance in your meals: include a variety of colors. Yes, colors. Add some green, yellow, red, orange, white, brown. The splashier the color display of your foods in their natural form, the more nutritional variety you have.

Try this with your salads, to start. You'll be surprised at the variety of tastes and textures you'll get with red cabbage, corn, carrots, and cooked pasta spirals added to your mixed salad greens, with a slice of dark bread on the side.

"Why go to all this trouble," you may ask, "when all I have to do is choose from the Basic Four food groups?" The Basic Four is fine as far as it goes, but it doesn't provide the information you need to choose wisely. The Basic Four can't tell the difference between a hot dog and a chicken breast, a sweet roll and a bowl of rice. Meat is meat and grain is grain.

Chances are your weight problem did not come about from not knowing the Basic Four, but rather, from not choosing the most nutrient-dense, low-fat, low-sugar choices.

Load Up With Complex Carbohydrates

Go ahead, pile your plate high with a variety of colorful, fresh vegetables on pasta or rice. Complex carbohydrates—such as whole grains, beans, fruits and vegetables—are the foundation of a healthful eating plan designed to fuel your body without adding fat. Add a small amount of protein in the form of lean meat, fish, poultry, or a vegetarian alternative such as tofu, and you've got a complete, balanced meal.

"Huh? Shouldn't I eat mostly protein?" you ask, remembering all those boring tuna fish and cottage cheese diets. You do need a small amount of protein at each meal, but most Americans eat much more than they need. Aim to get at least 60 percent of your calories as carbohydrates and about 10 percent as protein.

And here's another reason why you should increase your complex carbohydrates: they're rich in fiber, so they fill you up. You won't go hungry as you did on unsuccessful diets in the past. Since fiber-rich foods are filling and satisfying, you'll have an easier time saying "no" to fatty snacks and sugary desserts.

Misconceptions About Carbohydrates

The carbohydrates found in potatoes and pasta have been getting a bad rap for years. The truth is, they're not high in calories at all. And they're definitely not the fattening foods most people make them out to be. In fact, the body would rather burn than store them.

Carbohydrates, stored as glycogen in the liver and muscles, are the body's main source of energy. Pasta, bread, potatoes are all energy fuel. But be careful: if you cover the pasta with cream sauce and slather butter on the bread and potato, you're creating a high-fat monstrosity with double (or more) the calories. Turn those apples into apple pie, and the calories quadruple!

Try making the change to eating more complex carbohydrates at breakfast, when many of us do our high-fat eating. Instead of high-fat, high-protein bacon and eggs or high-fat, sugar-ladened sweet rolls, try a bowl of whole grain cereal with non-fat milk and fresh fruit. Your first surprise will be how tasty and filling this light meal can be. Your second surprise will be how many hours go by before you start to feel hungry again.

Be careful when choosing cereal, though. Read the package labels looking for whole grains—wheat or oats, for example—with a minimum of added sweeteners such as sugar, corn syrup, or any ingredient ending with "-ose."

Yes, supermarket shelves are filled with frosted, sugared, honeyed, and practically candied cereal choices. But most markets have plenty of more healthful alternatives, and health food stores offer even more. If you're used to sweetened cereals, fool your sweet tooth by adding a banana or a sprinkling of raisins, or both.

Be Patient: Results Are On The Way

When you choose well-balanced, nutritious meals that are high in carbohydrates, low in fat, and moderate in quantity, your body will start to change. But no one can predict how much nor how fast.

No one can guarantee that you'll lose x number of pounds in y days, or even that you'll lose x number of pounds at all. You'll see in a later chapter why this is impossible. But we can guarantee that your body will get leaner and you'll improve your quality of life.

Choosing the kind of eating plan we've outlined here will help your body and mind function at their peak levels. You'll feel healthier, more energetic and vigorous, and more productive. Your self-esteem will soar. Your lifestyle won't be limited by your body or your body image. And you'll be free from extreme dieting—forever.

Your Turn: How Well Are You Eating?

Go back and re-read the summary of the Four-day Eating Diary you prepared at the beginning of this chapter. Look at the information in terms of how well the foods you normally eat nourish your body.

1. Which of the foods you typically eat are high in nutrition?

2. Which foods are good quality, complex carbohydrates?

3. Which foods are high in fat, sugar, or are non-nutritious?

4. What changes would make your eating style more healthful and lower in fat?

5. What barriers do you expect to face when you start to change your eating habits?

6. What first step would you be willing to make, starting today?

One Step At A Time

By closely examining your eating lifestyle, you're beginning to see how your choices might be sabotaging your weight loss goals. Certain types of foods contribute to fat gain, others are used efficiently and cleanly by the body. One of the important keys to letting go of that excess fat is to alter your eating lifestyle when you recognize which habits keep you from losing weight.

They don't have to be drastic changes. We're not asking you to live on alfalfa sprouts and non-fat yogurt, or shop only in health food stores, or give up Thanksgiving dinner. You can still eat in restaurants without salad bars.

Your success depends on making lifestyle modifications that you can live with and feel better for having made them. This might mean taking a walk instead of eating your usual mid-morning doughnut. It might mean brown-bagging your lunch instead of heading for the fast food pit stop. Or ordering a baked potato instead of french fries. It might mean negotiating with your family for meatless meals a few days a week, or getting the ice cream out of the house.

The road to losing excess body fat is direct and clearly marked. True, the travel time might be long, and there are no short cuts or magic carpets. There are no free rides. Still, the voyage itself is pleasurable with much to discover along the way. And you get stronger each step of the way.

Liking yourself, respecting your decisions, taking an active role, feeling excited about the changes you're effecting—these all build on each other, pump you up and help you reach your goals. Take charge of your eating habits and get rid of the eating and non-exercising behavior that doesn't match the way you want to look.

Each change you make should be a positive, not a negative one. Rather than depriving yourself of something you like, look at it as taking you one step closer to having a leaner, healthier, more vibrant body.

You don't need to make all the changes at once. Take just one step at a time, just one day at a time. Adopting even one behavior change permanently will make a tremendous difference over time, as Jo discovered in the next case study.

Case Study: Jo

Jo, 46, identifies herself as a "recovering chocoholic." She gave up chocolate four years ago, after 20 years of eating it daily. "I'd drive miles out of my way to get the freshest chocolate chip cookies, or the highest quality truffles, then try not to eat them until after my aerobics class. At best, chocolate was a sensual experience. At worst, it was a craving."

Why did she give it up? "I finally realized that it didn't fit with the way I wanted to live my life or the way I wanted to see myself. I was a health-conscious, self-reliant person, enthusiastic about exercise and personal fitness. Where was my credibility if I'd go salivating after every single chocolate chip cookie?"

She tried to cut down, but that didn't work for her. So she decided to give up chocolate entirely. "I had to get the craving out of my system. I had to be as compulsive about not eating chocolate as I had been about eating it."

With just this one change, four pounds melted off the first month of chocolate abstinence and stayed off. "I didn't know I was eating that much of it!" Does she feel deprived? "Quite the contrary, I feel free. I don't think about it any more. My energy level is so much higher now that I'm not eating all that fat and sugar. I can watch everyone else eat chocolate and not even be tempted. I still like the smell, though."

7

Rating
The
Weight Loss Programs

The Good, The Bad, And The Useless

Now that you've decided to begin an eating program earmarked by low-fat, low-sugar consumption, you're faced with the $64,000 question: Are there diet plans and programs available that embrace this sensible nutritional advice, and are they compatible with your eating and exercising lifestyle?

The answer is an unequivocal YES!

But you have to sort through a virtual quagmire of competitive claims to find them. It may seem like a tedious exercise but finding the program that's right for your lifestyle is crucially important to your success. Here's why.

It's a proven fact: the more a potential weight loss plan runs counter to your present eating and activity lifestyle, the less likely your chances to lose weight permanently. The reasons why should be obvious. As dieting plans become more alien to your lifestyle, they become more difficult to stick to and, perhaps, more harmful to your health.

That's one of the big reasons why so many diet programs

are worth less than the paper they're printed on: they offer eating programs which are completely alien to most lifestyles.

For example, some overweight men and women are young, single, and living alone. They're much more likely to "eat on the run," to spend more time in social eating events involving other young people. In short, they're the last people you'd expect to lose weight using a diet that calls for spending considerable time in the kitchen working up recipes.

Contrast that with the average dieter. She's female, 42 years old, mother of one or two children, probably married. This woman has a totally different kind of lifestyle. Ms. Average Dieter might welcome the opportunity to spend considerable time kitchen-testing new low-calorie recipes but might resent eating one of those "milk shake" meals while the rest of her family enjoys a hearty pot roast.

In short, just as people come in infinite varieties, so too, are the eating plans that can match our lifestyles and give us the edge to achieving the thinner figures that we seek.

The charts that follow provide a handy comparison of some of the major features of leading weight loss programs. Inclusion on these pages is not meant as an endorsement. These weight loss plans are continually updating and adapting their programs, so investigate any changes since the publication of this book. And one additional word of caution: Remember to consult your physician before starting a diet or an exercise program.

An Endless Variety

We've investigated a wide variety of the plans and programs that are available to the man or woman who wants to lose weight. We studied the exchange diets, the programs that offer pre-packaged meal diets, the medically supervised "fasting" programs, diet aids such as diet shakes and low-fat, low-calorie frozen entrées, and support groups. And we've also read most of the diet books, those literary dieting entrées that glut the weight loss market.

Our most important finding is that there's something to recommend in many of these programs. Yes, there are still plenty of bizarre dieting plans out there that no nutritionist in his or her right mind would recommend. But if you shop carefully, you can find the plan that suits your eating lifestyle and reduces your weight.

How To Use This Guide

The sensible way to use this guide to help you select the one, right program is to keep in mind your exact goals:

1. Reduce fat consumption
2. Reduce sugar consumption
3. Match as closely as possible the eating behavior
   you can live with for the rest of your life

With this proviso in mind, let's move ahead with the Honest Truth.

Exchange Diets

Exchange diets don't count calories. Instead, you control your food intake by restricting the number of portions of meat protein, starch/bread, vegetable, fruit, dairy, and fat. You eat a prescribed number of exchanges, or servings, of each food group. Just remember your goals. And make any weight loss plan or program you use reduce dietary fat, sugar, and increase your level of exercise.

PROGRAM	FORMAT	DIET	COST
Diet Center	Daily counseling, progressive diet phases, group classes	Minimum 915 calories for women, 1255 for men 28% protein 47% carbohydrates 25% fat	Varies by pounds lost; approximately $700/30 lbs. in 8-9 weeks
Weight Watchers	Support group, variety of specialized meetings	25% protein 45% carbohydrates 30% fat	$12-20 for membership plus $8 a week

Pros:

Exchange diets teach nutritious eating habits while letting you make your own choices among "real" foods. You don't have to count calories and you generally get group support. They might be perfect for the person who has more time to cook and experiment with recipes, particularly the at-home mother.

Cons:

These programs might not have nutrition professionals available on a day-to-day basis, although the plans themselves have been developed by professionals. Your program is generally not individualized. There's no medical supervision.

Cautions:

Be careful not to confuse the Weight Watchers packaged foods with the Weight Watchers program. Read the labels: many have more than 30 percent in fat and are high in salt.

Pre-Packaged Meal Diets

Some weight loss centers offer pre-packaged, prepared meals. Join the program, buy meals, and lose the weight, they claim. Since you don't have to shop, cook, or make decisions, they might appeal to dieters whose lifestyles favor the "pre-packaged" format.

PROGRAM	DIET	COST
Jenny Craig	Minimum 950 calories women, 1100 men 20% protein 60% carbohydrates 20% fat	$185 membership plus $60-$70 a week for food
Nutri/System	1000-1500 calories 23% protein 61% carbohydrates 16% fat	Costs vary greatly. It can cost upwards of $750 to join, plus $60 a week for food.

Pros:

They're simple to understand and use because you eat only what they give you. Meals are well-balanced, portion- and calorie-controlled. You can use these programs even if you only have a few pounds to lose. A weight-maintenance plan is also included. Exercise is encouraged.

Cons:

Since the food is provided, you don't learn how to make your own shopping, cooking and eating decisions until after you lose your weight. You can't eat at restaurants or social gatherings while you're on the program. And because all food is processed, some nutrients are lost.

Classes are often taught by counselors with no background in nutrition. No medical supervision.

Cautions:

Check your calorie intake to make sure it isn't too low. It's difficult to get the nutrients you need at less than 1200 calories, and under 1,000 calories is not recommended without medical supervision. At this writing, Nutri/System faces lawsuits from dieters who allege that they developed gallstones from their low-calorie diets. Nutri/System denies all liability for their claims.

Liquid Diet Programs, Medically Supervised

These programs are actually semi-fasts. Instead of eating regular meals, you drink a liquid formula two to six times a day for 12-16 weeks, getting from 400 to 800 calories a day.

The second phase of these diets involves a gradual reintroduction of foods. Once you are eating all "real" foods again, you enter a maintenance phase where you learn to manage your weight while eating nutritiously.

PROGRAM	FORMULA	COST
HMR	800 calories 40% protein 49% carbohydrates 11% fat	$1300-$2775 depending on length of use
Medifast	435-848 calories 46-60% protein 28-41% carbohydrates 6-25% fat	$1700-$1900 for five months
Optifast	420-800 calories 67% protein 29% carbohydrates 4% fat	$2500-$3500 for 26 weeks

Pros:

If you're at least 30 percent or 50 pounds overweight and have medical conditions necessitating quick weight loss, these programs make the pounds come off quickly. Cholesterol, glucose, and triglyceride levels decrease. Blood pressure also drops.

Programs are administered in a hospital, clinic, or doctor's office, with medical attention weekly. The maintenance phase includes exercise and behavior modification programs.

Cons:

Since the weight loss is rapid, the initial loss is mostly water, then both fat and muscle, not just fat. Half the people who enroll in these programs don't stick around long enough to enter the maintenance phase, thereby setting themselves up for a weight gain almost as fast as the weight loss.

Moreover, your metabolic rate slows down, making weight regain likely after normal eating is resumed. The very low calorie intake reduces energy and exercise so that doing anything more energetic than mild walking is usually not recommended until the maintenance phase.

Calorie deprivation can lead to medical problems. Physicians working with these programs are often untrained in nutrition, body composition, and the physiological effects of severe calorie restriction.

These programs are also very costly. Long-term weight maintenance statistics are poor.

Cautions:

Use one of these programs only as a last resort and only if you are severely obese and your physician gives you medical reasons that warrant rapid weight loss. Check out the experience and qualifications of the medical staff and find out how much time you'll actually spend each week with a physician. Find out what kind of behavior modification program is offered, if any, because this is a crucial facet of making the program work.

Then, if you enroll in this kind of program, stick with it through the maintenance phase, which might involve a commitment of up to one year.

Over-The-Counter Diet Shakes

Just pop open a can and drink a 150-calorie meal. Or mix a scoop of powder with non-fat milk and drink your 220-calorie nutritionally balanced lunch. Or make a 70-calorie, creamy shake to stave off the urge to snack. Over-the-counter diet shakes are popular because these widely advertised confections are easy to use and are available in a variety of stores. And they've met with a fair degree of success because they favor busy, "no time to eat" lifestyles.

None of these products are intended to replace all food. If they appeal to you, use them only once or twice a day, and only when the remainder of your meals are nutritious, balanced, real food.

Pros:

For the busy, weight-conscious person on the go, using a diet shake as breakfast or lunch is convenient and simple.

Cons:

These diet "meals" are little more than sugared, flavored milk plus vitamins and minerals. The sweet taste might make you crave other sweet foods. Diet shakes don't have the "mouth feel" of real food, and could leave you dissatisfied.

DIET SHAKES	DESCRIPTION	COMMENTS
Alba '77	70-calorie snack shake not a meal. Mix with ice water.	Thick and creamy, good flavor Chemical aftertaste
Firmaloss	190 calories with non-fat milk	Less sweet tasting and more filling than most. Available in health food stores.
Naturade	200 calories with non-fat milk	Soy protein, high in protein and fiber, more filling than most
Sego	150-calorie liquid meal in a can	Main ingredients are milk and oil Chemical taste
SlimFast	190 calories with non-fat milk	Tastes like sugared milk; chemical aftertaste. Hunger recurs quickly.
Twinfast	80 calories with water High protein, low carbohydrate	Promotes dangerously low 800-calorie diet. Avoid this without medical supervision.
Ultra SlimFast	Slimfast with extra fiber 220 calories with low-fat milk	More filling than regular Slimfast Chemical aftertaste
Weigh Down	98 calories mixed with water or 198 calories with non-fat milk	Odd taste Advertises "Biochrome" as special ingredient

Many diet shakes have a chemical aftertaste. They're not as filling as the same number of calories in a large salad or non-fat milk plus fruit and cereal. You might feel hungry again within a couple of hours. They teach dependence on commercial products, instead of how to make lifestyle changes.

Cautions:

These products are fine as a quick convenience occasionally, but don't count on them for long-term weight control. Active exercisers might have trouble maintaining their energy level drinking these products instead of a meal. If you find these products limit the amount or intensity of exercise you can do, you're defeating the purpose of using them.

Don't accept at face value the claims you see in the ads or on the label. No food or special ingredient can raise metabolism (only exercise can do that), and it's doubtful that you'll feel full and satisfied with any of these products. Read the ingredients. You'll find sucrose (sugar) or fructose (fruit sugar) as a major ingredient. If you're trying to tame your sweet tooth, these won't help. Except where noted, the chart contains high carbohydrate powders to be mixed with nonfat milk as a replacement meal once or twice a day.

Low-fat, Low-Calorie Frozen Entrées

These new low-calorie main courses are not dieting programs, per se, but since they're used with growing frequency by dieters, we've included this section on "diet meals."

In the past, if you wanted a quick convenience dinner from the supermarket freezer, you had to sacrifice nutrition, your diet, and usually taste. Now several companies are giving us what we want: nutritious, low-fat frozen entrées that can provide guilt-free enjoyment. And they're tasty! The best of them don't even taste like diet foods.

Some Good Choices:

BRAND	CALORIES	FAT %	TYPE
Healthy Choice*	220-320	4-29%	Seafood, poultry, vegetarian, beef
Le Menu Light	220-310	7-26%	Poultry, vegetarian
Right Course	200-290	19-29%	Seafood, poultry, vegetarian, beef

* Judged "best tasting"

Pros:

Convenience, convenience, convenience, especially for the single person.

Cons:

If you're not careful in your choice, you can get a deceptively labeled, high-fat meal by mistake. Many brands were omitted from this list because they are high in sodium. Sodium is not only associated with high blood pressure and other bodily ills, but also predisposes your body to retain fluids, making your weight unnecessarily heavy.

They're more expensive than cooking from scratch, of course. Fresh ingredients are usually more nutritious than processed ingredients.

Cautions:

You have to use an eagle-eye and a hand-held calculator when trying to sort through these entrées, selecting good from not-so-good. The bad ones may say "light" (or "lite") and "lower" in fat, but if you do the fat/calorie calculation we described earlier, you might find that 40 to 50 percent of the calories come from fat. Don't believe the labels until you've done your own fat calculations.

Support Groups

Compulsive and binge eaters have a relationship to food that is similar to an alcoholic's relationship to alcohol. Once they start eating, they can't seem to stop. They have an obsessive relationship with food and eat more for psychological reasons than for physical hunger.

Compulsive eating is a way of life for some people, or an occasional problem for others. It might be triggered by certain foods, times of day, or stressful situations.

Compulsive eaters often feel secretive and alone. Joining others with the same problem can help an overeater look at the reasons for the behavior and learn skills for overcoming it. Again, look first to your lifestyle and see if a support group might not be just what you need.

PROGRAM	FORMAT	COST
Overeaters Anonymous	Support group, similar to AA, for compulsive overeaters	Voluntary contributions
TOPS (Take Off Pounds Sensibly)	Support group, similar to AA, weekly meetings	$12 year

To Join Or Not . . .

Should you join a program to help you change your eating habits? That depends. If you're looking for salvation, an easy fix, or weight loss magic, you will probably find the programs wanting. Such a program doesn't exist.

Adopting the habits that get and keep weight off takes motivation, concentration and commitment. You've got to want to do what it takes—not just get the results. Any program that claims to do all the work for you is lying to you and will lighten only your wallet.

But if you're willing to learn about nutrition and exercise and make a commitment to change behavior, and if you don't want to do this alone, a program may help. Some programs sell meals, others offer menu lists, some give support. Investigate the possibilities thoroughly. Don't make a choice based only on a friend's weight loss or a magazine ad.

Many people like the pre-packaged diet plans or prepared menus that some programs offer. It's easy to eat correctly because you don't have to figure out your own balanced, low-fat, low-calorie meals. With some, you don't even have to step into a grocery store. The decision-making isn't up to you.

That's good and bad. It's good because it's convenient, and you're more apt to stick with it. It's bad because it doesn't teach you to make your own healthful, appropriate choices. Remember, these are *lifelong* eating changes, not short-term dieting panaceas. Sooner or later you'll want or need to prepare your own meals with your own preferences, without regaining your weight. Will you know how?

If the convenience seems like a lifeline right now, you might like to join a pre-packaged or prepared menu program for just a short time, while you learn about low-fat cooking and healthful eating choices. Choose one with a registered dietician on staff. (Note that anyone can call herself or himself a nutritionist, but a registered dietician must have a degree in nutrition, pass a state examination, and keep current with continuing education.) Find out what sort of training the program's counselors have.

You can get a motivational spurt from the camaraderie of a weight control support group. Weight Watchers, Overeaters Anonymous and TOPS (Take Off Pounds Sensibly) are the best known. Support groups don't sell food, although some offer recommended menus or exchange lists. Most important is the feeling of commitment to the group and the sharing of personal issues, and the focus on behavioral changes.

Finding The Bookstore Diet That Fits Your Lifestyle

Bookstore diets present the same problem as the other diet programs. You have to wade through the hundreds of programs to find the one features food and plans that fit your eating and activity lifestyles. Here's how to start your analysis of bookstore diets:

1. Look first at the plan itself: Is it medically safe and nutritionally sound? Does it offer weight loss ideas that are backed by major medical authorities?
2. Is the eating plan compatible with your lifestyle? Does the diet plan suggest spending hours in the kitchen but you're an eat-and-run personality? Does it suggest you eat foods that are totally unlike your eating history?
3. Is it a plan you can life with—the rest of your life? Sure you can eat grapefruit and lemons for a day, or maybe even a week. But can you live on a grapefruit diet the rest of your life? Of course not, so don't bother trying it in the first place.

With these provisos, let's look at what bookstore bestsellers are offering these days.

The Fit Or Fat Target Diet by Covert Bailey

Bailey's work is probably the most important work on the weight loss book shelf that you're likely to find, since he shows how to plan a sensible low-fat diet that reduces calories and increases exercise.

To that end, Bailey omits all those diet menus that bulk up most diet books. He stresses instead a 1,200 calorie diet for women using the Four Food Groups' recommendations.

Bailey also presents a unique system for analyzing diets (yours or anyone else's). His recommendations are what you'd hear from any knowledgeable dietician or health-care professional: Get a handle on how much fat you eat and how much you exercise, and the weight reduction will take care of itself.

Recommendations: Here's a book that will work well in your effort to start with the basics: low-fat and more exercise. From there, it's easy to use Bailey's plan for establishing an on-going eating plan that fits your lifestyle. Use this book, along with ours, and you can be a winner!

The Rotation Diet by Martin Katahn, Ph.D.

Katahn believes that you can lose weight more easily and quickly if you can avoid the metabolic slowdown that often accompanies diets, a phenomenon we noted earlier. His solution, heavily promoted in a well-orchestrated media blitz, is to "rotate" the diet during a three-week program.

His program allows 600 calories for three days, 900 calories for four days, and then 1,200 calories a day for one week, after which you again rotate the 600 and 900 calories.

It doesn't take a dietician to recognize the shortfall here.

Any diet than recommends 600 and 900 calories a day is substantially below dieticians' recommendations. Moreover, Katahn offers scant clinical evidence that his program works. Indeed, the American Journal of Clinical Nutrition said the type of caloric restriction proposed by this type of diet does not affect weight or fat loss.

Recommendations: We think Katahn's promises outweigh documented results. There's not a single dietician we know who would recommend 600 or 900 calories a day and there's no proof this plan works any better than traditional weight loss programs. We say skip this one.

The Pritikin Permanent
Weight-Loss Manual by Nathan Pritikin

Pritikin is the man whose name is synonymous with the low-cholesterol, high-complex carbohydrate diet, the same Pritikin whose Longevity Center is famous for helping patients suffering from degenerative diseases.

The manual offers four food plans: 1,200, 1,000, 850, and 700 calories. Each contains menus reasonably well-balanced in nutrients. The problem is that Pritikin's menus are pretty strict. Fat allowances in his programs, for example, amount to only 10 percent. That's 20 percent below what the American Heart Association targets for the American diet.

Recommendations: Overall, Pritikin's weight loss program is on target. You'll likely face considerable problem in sticking to his 10 percent fat recommendation, though. But for dieters who strike a balance, his plan is among the best. We'd say skip the extremely low-calorie plans and go for 1,200 calories a day. P.S.: Trust Pritikin when he says a systematic program of exercise is crucial to weight loss success.

Elizabeth Takes Off by Elizabeth Taylor

Question: Would you trust a diet cooked up by someone who is arguably one of the world's champion "yo-yo" dieters? Answer: Don't do as I do—do as I say. And Liz says plenty, even though much of it has been said before.

Liz's program, for example, is mostly a 1970s "high-protein, low-carbohydrate" diet retrofitted with her personal account of what it's like to balloon from screen goddess to the butt of Hollywood pundits.

Recommendations: Liz's book makes interesting reading, particularly those who want more than a healthful serving of Hollywood glitterati. It might be especially helpful to dieters needing a program to help them win back their self-image and self-esteem. Though much of her advice is sound, her plan is too heavily weighted to protein, and not enough complex carbohydrates.

**Dr. Berger's Immune
Power Diet** by Stuart M. Berger, M.D.

If you have a penchant for the bizarre, Berger is your man. Berger's three-phase "immune" diet promises "important and lasting weight loss where other diets have failed." What you get is what Berger calls a 21-day "Elimination Diet" during which you're not to eat the same food more than once every four days, a 14-day reintroduction plan; and a followup maintenance plan.

Like most of the diet plans of its type, Berger includes lot of recipes—many of them more suitable to Himalayan monk than your average dieter (carrot puree on a bed of leeks, for example). Berger recognizes that his plan is controversial but says it's been tried and proven effective with 3,000 of his patients.

Recommendations: Berger's plan is medically flimsy and likely to stray too far afield of most dieters' eating lifestyles. But don't take our word for it. Jean Mayer, Ph.D., Sc.D., a noted nutritionists and president of Tufts University where Berger received his medical training, said of the diet: "It is my hope that no future graduate of the Tufts medical school will exhibit as little knowledge of nutrition as does Mr. Berger in this book."

The 8-Week Cholesterol Cure by Robert E. Kowalski

Kowalski is a medical writer who devised this program as a way to reduce his cholesterol program after other methods had failed him. Kowalski says he tried the other cholesterol-reducing food plans, including those from the American Heart Association, Pritikin, even drugs.

His plan is not exactly a weight-reducing "diet." Kowalski's program features a diet which is low in fat, high in complex carbohydrates; which, he says, dropped his blood cholesterol levels from 284 to 169.

Recommendations: The low-fat, high complex carbohydrate portions of Kowalski's plan are good. And for that reasons, we can suggest that it could have a part in your food planning. But watch out for Kowalski's prescription of megadoses of niacin. Medical reports say such doses could pose serious side effects, including irregular heart beats and liver damage.

Your Program Check List

Good weight loss programs teach you an eating lifestyle you can follow for life. They do all of the following:

✓ Teach balance, variety, and moderation

✓ Individualize weight loss goals and calorie intake

✓ Provide or recommend enough calories to maintain good health

✓ Teach you to make your own healthful choices

✓ Promote weight loss of no more than 1-2 pounds a week

✓ Follow dietary guidelines for sound nutrition

✓ Help you make changes in your behavior

✓ Encourage a balanced fitness program with both strength and aerobic exercise for weight loss and maintenance

✓ Offer a thorough maintenance program after goal weight is achieved

✓ Allow food that makes you feel satisfied, not deprived

✓ Emphasize meals low in fat, high in complex carbohydrates, and moderate in protein

Seven Honest Truths
About
Diets And Weight Loss

1. Permanent fat loss is only possible with a slow, steady, safe, and sensible eating plan.

2. Extreme diets are never a permanent answer and could be dangerous.

3. When you put less fat into your mouth, you will reduce the amount of fat you carry on your body.

4. To control your weight, you'll need to find a life-time eating plan (not a temporary diet) that's low in fat and high in nutrition, complex carbohydrates and variety.

5. Personalizing your eating plan so that it suits your taste and your lifestyle will move you consistently towards your goals.

6. Tracking your program with a tape measure provides the motivation you need to achieve weight loss success.

7. Strong motivation is the key to losing weight permanently. Be good to yourself and take credit for your success.

Part II

The Honest Truth

About Exercise

And

Permanent Weight Loss

8

Exercise: The Key
To Permanent Fat Loss

The wise, for cure, on exercise depend.
—**John Dryden (1631-1700)**

Exercise: Your Fat Furnace

Inevitably, people who lose weight solely through caloric restrictions regain it. The folks who keep their pounds off do it by a sensible, low-fat, low-sugar diet with a regular program of exercise. Why does that happen?

For one thing, people who exercise naturally increase their metabolic rate and that makes sustained weight loss infinitely easier. Let's take a closer look at what that means.

Even at rest, your body is hard at work, keeping all its systems running. Your heart, lungs, digestive system and all the other inner workings don't rest while you catch some shut-eye. The functioning of all those systems—called metabolism—requires energy, which the body gets by converting food into glucose, the body's fuel.

Calories are the measure of the amount of energy supplied by food and used in metabolism. The rate at which this happens is called the metabolic rate. Put more simply, your metabolic rate is how fast your body burns calories. Your basal metabolic rate measures your body's calorie-burning at rest.

The Genes And Metabolism

Each of us has a different metabolic rate that is apparently genetically determined. People with higher metabolic rates have an easier time managing their weight because they burn calories faster. Those of us with slower metabolic rates may eat no more than our skinny friends, yet still we put on weight.

No, it's not fair, but there's little we can do to recast our hereditary fate. There is one sure, powerful way we can stoke the fat-burning furnace and raise our metabolic rate: exercise. Exercise is essential for making long-term weight changes.

Here's why. First of all, exercise burns calories. For each mile you walk, for every minute of aerobic dance, for every stride on your NordicTrack, your body burns more fuel. All things considered equal, if our food intake remains constant, then any extra exercise will burn calories by drawing from our stored fat.

This happy event produces a double bonus:

(1) We stop putting on extra fat; and
(2) We start burning off all that unwanted fat.

But there's much more to the story than the *quid pro quo* whereby one unit of added exercise produces one unit of lost weight. Exercise speeds up the loss of body fat by *raising your metabolic rate*. Exercise also increases your body's proportion of active, calorie-hungry, lean tissue. Each workout stokes your fat furnace, making it burn and use fuel more quickly. The result: you get thinner, faster, easier. And what could be better than that?

The Myth Of Spot Reducing

Sorry, there's no such thing as spot reducing. Where we carry our fat is genetically determined. Working specific muscles will strengthen and shape them, but won't get rid of fat in a localized area.

Generally, the toughest places to lose fat are exactly those places we want to slim down most: the abdomen (men and women), buttocks and thighs (women). No number of curl-ups or sit-ups will reduce the abdominal fat—though they will certainly help tone and shape that area. If you've got a fat belly and you do 10 minutes of curl-ups a day, you'll have strong, toned muscles, but they'll be hidden under the fat.

The solution? Exercise aerobically to reduce body fat, and do those curl-ups and other muscle-specific exercises for toning and strengthening. Aerobic exercise burns fat from all over our body, slimming down our trouble spots as well, and body toning work will help give those areas a defined, more sleek appearance.

More Important Benefits From Exercise

A well-chosen fitness program offers even more than a neat, easy way to lose weight. It also helps you perform better in your daily life. Human beings are meant to move. If you sit or stand in one position most of the day, you can't help feeling stiff, tired, and eventually, less productive.

The right exercise program will help your posture and decrease fatigue. A fitness program that emphasizes the muscles you don't use at work will help you balance your body and reduce tension at the end of the day. Use exercise to revitalize your mind, and stretch to relieve the stiffness.

The Crucial Need For Balanced Fitness

What do you want from your exercise program? Sure, you

want to lose weight. But what else? Are you looking for improvements in your health? In your body shape? Would you like to increase your stamina? Get stronger? More flexible? Interact with other people? Reduce stress? Whatever your exercise goals, a program of balanced fitness—the combination of regular aerobic exercise with strength training—will help you reach them.

Balanced fitness is also about moderation. You don't have to become a gung-ho athlete to achieve all of the above. You don't have to run marathons, win tennis matches, or even walk a twelve-minute mile. The key is consistency and frequency, not intensity. You're competing with no one, except, perhaps, yourself. You're pushing towards your own potential, minute by minute, day by day.

Here's How Exercise Can Work Wonders For You!

Helene, 65 and vibrant, has used exercise and low-fat eating to bring her high cholesterol count down to normal. She works out regularly at a health club, combining low-impact aerobics and strength training, and keeps physically active through gardening and other interests. Her body is tight and strong, and she looks fitter than most women half her age.

Donna, 44, was 40 pounds overweight as a teenager, and gained 20 pounds more in her thirties. She could always lose weight dieting but inevitably gained it back. On her fortieth birthday, her family presented her with a NordicTrack cross-country ski machine. Though she didn't have much stamina at first, she liked the way exercising made her feel. She stuck with it, lost her weight gradually over six months, and kept the weight off.

"I started out exercising just to lose weight, but now I do it because I love it. The weight control is a great side benefit of doing something I enjoy."

Carl, 32, used to be 100 pounds overweight. "In the summer, my pants would rub together. I'd get too hot to walk more than a couple of blocks because my legs would get so warm from rubbing. I used to get rashes."

He started a program of balanced, low-fat eating and regular exercise, and discovered he enjoyed sports. Then a woman friend dared him to try her sport, aerobic dance. Though he felt uncoordinated and clumsy at first, he enjoyed working out to music in a group and continued to attend. Now his body is trim and muscled, and Carl is an aerobics instructor who delights in motivating his students.

Helene, Donna and Carl have much in common, despite differences in age, gender and background:

1. They had weight or health problems that led to their starting an exercise program.
2. They made permanent reductions in their body fat.
3. They reshaped their bodies.
4. They permanently adopted a physically active lifestyle.
5. They exercise for the pleasure of it.

Pushing Through The Plateau

Sometimes, weight loss programs seem to run into a dead end. The scale stops dead in its tracks. No amount of exercising or caloric restriction seems to get it moving downward.

Sally, 41, is a good example. She had been riding her exercise bicycle faithfully for 35 minutes every other morning for a year. She liked the way it pepped her up and was delighted at how it was slimming her down. Then suddenly her weight loss plateaued.

"It was as if my body said, 'Okay, I'm used to this exercise and I'm comfortable with this weight.' But I still had a dress size to go to meet my goal." Sally started alternating her exercise bike workouts with a stimulating workout on a cross-country ski-exerciser. Soon she was losing inches again. "And my legs, arms, shoulders and buttocks got much stronger and more shapely!"

Has your weight loss skidded to a halt, even though you're exercising several hours a week? Again, remember balance is the key. Try varying your exercise routine with the great variety of in-home or club exercise equipment available. Your body might have adapted to your workout and be signaling the need for a change. If you continue to push yourself harder without varying your activity, you risk injury as well as disappointment. Try switching to an entirely different activity on alternate days. You'll again start making progress in both weight loss and fitness.

Balancing Life

Elaine, 34, a computer programmer, always enjoyed her job, except that it kept her hunched over a keyboard most of the day. By the time she left work, her shoulders, back and neck ached. Soon Elaine realized that taking a short break on her Nordic Fitness Chair was a simple solution. It provided a complementary group of exercises that relieved her stress and stretched out those tired muscles.

Adding physical activity to your daily life will decrease fatigue and improve your stamina. There is a variety of ways you can increase your activity level. For example, at work, take a "stress break" with a Nordic Fitness Chair or an Executive Power Chair. Take the stairs instead of the elevator. Park near the exit instead of close to the stores in the shopping center. Get off the bus a few stops from your destination and

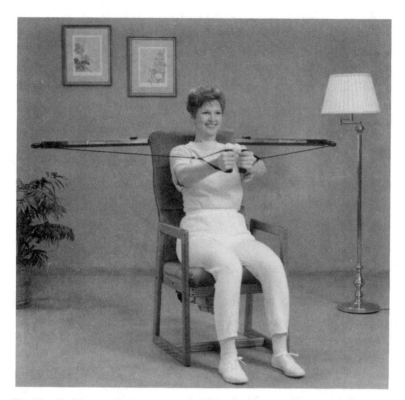

The Nordic Fitness Chair uses isokinetic resistance, the medically preferred method of strengthening muscles. Stronger muscles create a greater caloric burn to help achieve weight loss goals. Shown is the new Éclat model. (Photo courtesy of NordicTrack)

walk the rest of the way. Shovel snow, mow the lawn, rake leaves, chop firewood. And involve the rest of the family—especially the kids—in outings centered on physical activity. Balance: it's the cornerstone of a solid, satisfying life.

Creating Your Fat-Burning Machine

Why not start creating your own fat-burning machine with exercise? The chief component of your machine will be aerobic exercise. We'll discuss aerobic exercise more fully in the next chapter but for now, remember that aerobic exercise burns fat, strengthens you heart, and gives you energy and vitality. We want to look good and feel healthy and vigorous. To function well, we also need enough strength and flexibility to do the activities that are part of our lifestyle—and to keep doing them as we get older.

We can't get all these fitness components from any one type of exercise. To keep us active, healthy, strong, flexible and lean, we need a balanced program that delivers more than any one exercise alone.

Does this mean you have to exercise three hours instead of one to fit everything in? Not at all. If you choose activities that complement each other, you'll need less, not more, workout time. That's because you're exercising more efficiently and getting a greater return on your fitness investment. Balanced fitness will give you more time in your day, not take it away.

When you have all three, aerobic exercise, strength training, and flexibility, you're in shape and ready to carve out the all-important weight loss benefits that raising your metabolic rate can offer.

The Importance Of Stretching

> *The point of exercise is not just to lose weight, but to get back in touch with your body and enjoy physical exertion for its own sake. Fitness is one of the easiest things a person can have. It doesn't take any talent. All you're trying to do is develop your own potential.*
> **—Bob Anderson, author of *Stretching***

Stretching is important for keeping our bodies flexible, preventing injury, and maintaining a range of motion. Stretching also aids your exercise program by relaxing the muscles after you work them, rather than leaving muscles in a tight, contracted, uncomfortable state.

For best results, finish each exercise session with 10 minutes of stretching, more if you enjoy it. After a tense day, loosen up with 5 minutes of rhythmic warm-up, then indulge in 15 or more minutes of relaxing stretches.

To stretch a muscle effectively, use slow, static stretches, by relaxing into the stretch, breathing deeply, sinking a little farther each time you exhale. Avoid "ballistic" stretches which use fast, forceful, jerky, or bouncy motions. These do no good because the muscles react to sudden, exaggerated stretching by tightening instead of relaxing. Never force a stretch beyond your comfortable limit. Avoid any motion that puts stress on the knees, neck or back. To learn more about stretching, get a good book, videotape, or take a class.

Commit To Fitness

It's a simple fact:

**Exercise must be part of your lifestyle
if you want to keep your body fat low.**

If you're not an exerciser, those words might seem like a prison sentence. In fact, it's the opposite: exercise is an open gate to freedom. Feeling the joy of movement—feeling your body respond with power, rhythm and grace—all this comes with physical exertion.

No, it's not too late to get back in shape. Yes, it will take work. But if you'll make a commitment to regular exercise, you can strengthen your heart while conditioning and shaping your body, and you'll enjoy it more than you think.

The trick is to look at what you want exercise to accomplish for you personally. Then choose a workout you enjoy that will help you meet your goals.

Select your exercises as carefully as you choose your food and friends, and choose exercise that won't stress your joints or weakened areas. Be an aware fitness consumer.

Barney, 65, fit and spry, waves to a friend while riding the exercise bicycle at the health club. He usually bicycles outside, but it is raining today. He used to run regularly, but his knees can't take the stress now, so he bikes every day for aerobic exercise and then uses a NordicPower to keep his muscles strong and flexible.

What keeps him exercising? "Quality of life," he says with a smile. "I used to be a blob. Now I'm in pretty good shape. And really, my life has been all the better for it."

Don't Wait!

Maybe you've been saying, "I'll start an exercise program after I've lost some weight." Do you recognize how this plan is backwards?

Exercise keeps your body young, your mind alert, your energy high, your stress level low—and your sense of play alive. It complements and enriches the other parts of your life and helps you live fully and exhuberantly.   Moving with grace, power and pleasure is not the exclusive domain of the lean. Start now.

Your Turn: Your Exercise Habits And Preferences

Good, you've made your decision: it's time to put exercise back in your life. Here or in your private notebook, write your answers to these questions. They will help you start an exercise program by choosing activities that you'll really enjoy. If you already have an exercise program, these questions will help you make changes so that you enjoy it more.

1. Think back to the physical activities you used to enjoy as a child or teenager. Recall not only what you did, but how you felt while doing those activities. Write them down:

2. What physical activities have you done as an adult? What exercise activities do you do now? Include how many minutes per week you normally spend on each one.

3. How much do you enjoy your present exercise pattern? If you don't enjoy it, what could you change so that you do?

4. Did you ever exercise regularly? If so, what did you do, and why did you quit? If you decided to start again, would you do the same activity or try something else?

5. List two to five kinds of exercise that would fit your preferences and your schedule. Circle the one you want to try right away. What do you need to do to prepare?

9

Aerobic Exercise:
Your Fat Meltdown

Aerobic exercise is by far the most important part of weight control.

—**Covert Bailey,** *The Fit or Fat Woman*

What Is Aerobic Exercise?

Aerobic exercise is sustained, rhythmic movement using the large muscle groups, such as the thighs, buttocks, calves, and back. Aerobic exercise raises your heart rate and body temperature, and makes you perspire comfortably, given normal environmental conditions. It makes you breathe harder, but should not leave you winded or ever take you to the point of pain.

Aerobic exercise is absolutely the best gift you can give to yourself, to your weight loss program. As we said before: people who make exercise a habit manage to lose body fat and don't regain it. People who lose weight from diet alone almost always regain it. And the most important kind of exercise for decreasing body fat is aerobic. It's also the best gift you can give your body's most important muscle: the heart.

Aerobic exercise elevates your heart rate comfortably, it

does not leave you panting and lying in a puddle of your own sweat. Many exercisers, in fact, report a feeling of well-being, even euphoria, as their bodies hit their stride. If you're winded, dizzy, red-faced, or gasping, you're driving yourself much too hard.

Here are some examples of aerobic activities. Which is the best? The activity you will actually do. Give yourself a variety that you'll enjoy.

OUTDOOR	CLUB OR CLASS	HOME
jogging	aerobic dancing	ski-exerciser
brisk walking	fast ballroom dancing	rowing machine
bicycling	square dancing	exercise bike
cross-country skiing	step/bench classes	exercise videos
swimming	full court basketball	stair climbing
hill hiking	jazz dancing	treadmill
skating	aqua aerobic class	jumping rope
water running	interval training	jumping jacks
soccer	aerobic machines	jogging in place

If you're active in your home or leisure life, you might be getting some aerobic exercise already. Mowing the lawn can be aerobic, especially if you have a big lawn. Likewise, digging the garden, washing windows, raking leaves, and similar activities can fire up your aerobic fat-burning fires.

As long as your activity is rhythmic and continuous, uses the large muscles, and makes you perspire, it's aerobic, even if you do it to shape up your yard, not your body.

How Does Aerobic Exercise Help Me Lose Fat?

You've probably seen the charts that tell how many calories various activities burn per minute. You may have looked up your favorite exercise and found that it burns seven to eight calories per minute. All that work just to burn off one large apple with 20 minutes of exercise?

Let's look closer. Eight calories a minute times 20 minutes is 120 calories burned. Do that every day and you burn 840 calories a week, or a hefty 43,680 calories a year. That's 12-1/2 pounds lost through just 20 minutes a day!

ACTIVITY	CALORIE EXPENDITURE*
Bicycling	250-450
Bowling	100-190
Calisthenics	150-350
Cross-country skiing	660-1000
Downhill skiing	200-450
Golf	100-225
Handball & Racquetball	300-700
Housework	100-150
Office work	100-150
Rowing	660-900
Running	450-850
Skating (Ice or Roller)	300-520
Swimming	250-370
Walking	200-350

*Calories burned per hour. Lower figures are for women, higher numbers are for vigorous workouts by men. The heavier you are, the more vigorous the workout, the more calories you burn.

Even better, the fat-burning power doesn't end when you finish your workout. Aerobic exercise is the accelerator that makes your fat-burning engine work harder and faster for hours. Now that's as close to magic as you'll find!

Maybe you burned eight calories a minute while you were exercising (though the exact number is individual, and a chart only gives you an approximation). But the real reason aerobic exercise rules the kingdom of lost inches is its ability to raise your metabolic rate and keep it raised for hours after your exercise session has ended. That means you burn calories at a faster rate even as you go about your daily life.

Finding The Time

We can all find 20 minutes somewhere in our day to exercise. For maximum fat-burning, though, try to exercise aerobically for more than 20 minutes. Not only do you burn more calories, but you get a benefit you can't get any other way: you start consuming your fat stores. Scientists have found that if you continue to exercise aerobically past 20 minutes, you burn stored fat as fuel.

Yes, aerobic exercise will melt away buttock puckers, pooched-out bellies, and drooping upper arm fat.

For optimum fat burning, stay in your target range for 30 minutes or more, at least three times a week—more often if you can. Physiologists say that 40-plus minutes, four or more times a week, is even better, but please don't use that intimidating number as an excuse to throw your tennies back in the closet. The fact is: doing any aerobic exercise is far better for your health, your heart, your sense of well-being, and your weight loss than doing none at all.

Give up that all-or-nothing approach. You know how that ends: "all" the first week, and "nothing" after that. Instead, work into exercise easily. Do just five minutes if that's all you can do comfortably, then five more minutes later in the day, and maybe another five minutes in the evening. If the total is at least 20 minutes, even if you have to space them out, you get many of the benefits.

Keep at it consistently, and you'll find your stamina improves quickly. Soon you're able to do more than you thought possible. If you make regular aerobic exercise a habit, your body gets used to it, and it's easier to hit your stride and stay in your comfort zone for longer. Your body also gets used to revving up its metabolic rate. Not only do you burn calories faster than before, you maintain your weight loss with little effort.

Of course, if you have any physical limitations or medical conditions, check with your physician. Likewise if you're on medications find out how they affect your heart rate and what intensity is right for you. Your physician will probably be pleased that you want to start exercising, but he or she might have some cautions particular to your health status.

Hitting The Target:

Making Aerobic Exercise Pay Off

To make your exercise aerobic, aim to elevate your heart rate to 60-85 percent of maximum exertion and keep it there. This is called the "target heart rate range," and there are formulas and charts available to help you find yours. The most common method is to take your age, subtract it from 220, and then multiply by 60 and 85 percent. For example, if you're forty years old, you'd take 220 - 40 and get 180. Multiply by the 60-85 percentage and your target heart range for exercise is between 108 and 153 heart beats per minute.

For a more accurate, personalized target heart range, fill in the blanks on the following chart using the Karvonen formula. Start by taking your resting heart rate when you first wake up in the morning, before you get out of bed. Put two fingers on your pulse at your neck or wrist and count the beats for a full 30 seconds, and then double that figure to get your resting heart rate for one minute.

When you're exercising, your target range is the zone between the low end of your target rate, and the high end of your target rate. Take your pulse frequently during exercise

KARVONEN FORMULA

220
−_____ your age
=_____ maximum heart rate
−_____ resting heart rate
=_____
x__.60____ exercise intensity level
=_____
+_____ resting heart rate
=_____ **low end of your target rate**

220
−_____ your age
=_____ maximum heart rate
−_____ resting heart rate
=_____
x__.85____ exercise intensity level
=_____
+_____ resting heart rate
=_____ **high end of your target rate**

• The Institute for Aerobics Research recommends a target heart rate zone (THRZ) of 65-80 percent of your maximal heart rate.

• The American Heart Association recommends a THRZ of 60-75 percent of your maximal heart rate.

• The American College of Sports Medicine suggests a THRZ of 65-90 percent of your maximal heart rate.

to make sure you're hitting your target. To see if you're exercising aerobically, take your pulse for 10 seconds and multiply by six. If you're below your target rate, add intensity. Above it, you're working too hard. If aerobic exercise is your game, stay in the target range.

To step up the fat-burning process, exercise longer or more often, *but not harder*. If you get above your target heart rate, you're defeating your fat-loss purpose since you'll be unable to keep exercising. You'll also be more prone to muscle aches and injuries.

So take it cool. Pace yourself for longer workouts by staying in your low to moderate target heart range, and watch the fat melt away over time.

The simplest way to get a rough estimate of whether you're exercising within your target heart range is to monitor your body signals. If you match all of the following signs, you're exercising in your target range:

- You're feeling warm from the exertion
- You're perspiring comfortably
- Your heart is beating faster, but you don't feel winded
- You're breathing a little harder, but you can still talk in full sentences without gasping

If you can't talk or breathe easily, you feel weak, or you're fighting to keep moving, you're working too hard and defeating your purpose. Lower your intensity by moving slower or taking a break. Don't just stop cold, though. Walk in place or sit down and keep moving the arms and legs slowly. Keep your head above the level of your heart until your breathing is back to normal. You'll need to take your pulse at rest, and then take your pulse frequently during exercise to see if you're hitting your target.

Starting Your In-Home
Aerobic Exercise Program

There's a variety of quality, in-home exercise equipment available to help you build aerobic conditioning. For example, equipment like the NordicTrack and NordicRow TBX maximize aerobic conditioning because they involve all major upper and lower body muscle groups.

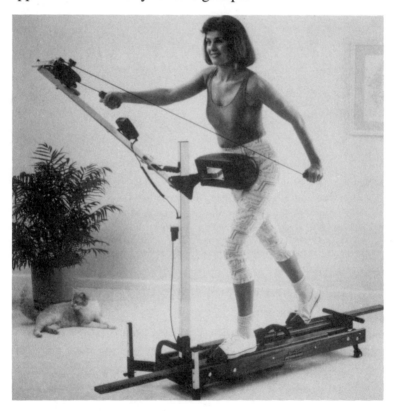

NordicTrack duplicates the total-body motion of cross-country skiing, and burns more calories than other forms of aerobic exercise. It provides a complete cardiovascular workout as well as complete upper- and lower body conditioning. (Photo courtesy of NordicTrack)

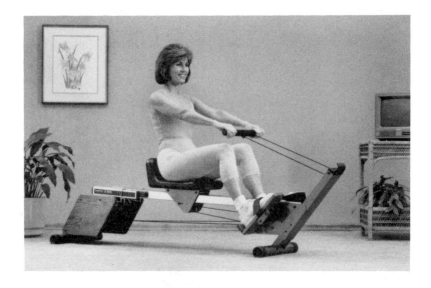

The NordicRow TBX gives dieters a total body workout. Separate upper and lower body resistance settings allow users to tailor their workouts to their particular level of fitness. Its manufacturers say a 20-minute workout, three times a week, will strengthen, burn fat, and improve cardiovascular fitness. (Photo courtesy of NordicTrack)

Your Turn: Which Aerobic Exercises Are For You?

1. List all the kinds of aerobic exercise that you have done as an adult. Refer to our exercise chart on an earlier page to refresh your memory. Put a check in front of those you do regularly now.

2. List all the kinds of aerobic exercise that you are interested in doing. Be specific. Write "take a beginning jazz dance class" rather than just "dance," for example.

3. What do you need to get started? (Examples: buy walking shoes, buy a cross-country ski exerciser, join a club, look in the newspaper for a class beginning soon, etc.)

4. Choose one familiar aerobic activity and a new one that you're willing to try on a regular basis for six weeks. Write them here:

Familiar Activity   **New Activity**

10

Strength Training: Getting Strong, Staying Lean

Lean muscle mass is your metabolic engine.

—Cardiologist James Rippe, M.D., University of Massachusetts

What Is Strength Training?

Strength training is the principle of making muscle stronger through a program of exercises that overload specific muscle groups. And it literally works miracles when it comes to losing weight. Here's why.

Remember how depressing it was to learn that extreme dieting actually slowed down your metabolic rate and made your body cling to its meager calorie intake? Here's the lighter side. Muscle is active tissue, and it demands more calories than fat just to maintain itself.

Think of muscle as similar to a hungry teenage boy: eating constantly, always active, growing bigger and stronger, but staying lean. The muscle in your body uses more calories even at rest than your fat. So it makes sense that the more lean tissue and less body fat you have, the higher your metabolic rate, and the faster you burn calories. Muscle makes your body a lean, calorie-burning machine.

For example, Anne and Sarah are each 5'4" tall and weigh 140 pounds. Anne strength trains. Sarah does not. Therefore, Anne's 140 pound body has more lean muscle than Sarah's. When they take a brisk, four-mile walk, Anne burns more calories than Sarah. If they eat the same meal afterwards, Sarah will store more of her calories as fat than Anne.

> **Research shows that every pound of fat we replace with muscle raises our metabolic rate by about 50 calories a day.**

Likewise, every pound of muscle we lose lowers it by the same amount. So a person on a strength training program will burn more calories per day than a person who eats the same amount but doesn't strength train, even if they both do the same aerobic workout.

Improved strength also helps you lead a physically active lifestyle with more energy and less risk of injury. This helps you in all parts of your life, not just your exercise hours. You'll carry kids, golf clubs and groceries without back strain, climb stairs without huffing and puffing, and pull your suitcases out of the car without wrenching your shoulder. And you'll feel more powerful and have more energy throughout the day.

How Strength Training Works

According to the Institute for Aerobics Research, muscles grow stronger in response to overload or stress.This stress can be accomplished in four ways:

1. Increasing resistance
2. Increasing repetitions
3. Decreasing rest time between repetitions
4. Increasing the number of training sessions
   each week

What really happens in strength training is that by over-loading a muscle, it is moderately damaged. To protect against future damage, the muscle grows stronger.

At first, you might not even need weights or resistance other than your own body. As you get fitter, you'll need more resistance—meaning a prop that you pull, push, or lift against to make the muscles work harder.

For example, when you're first getting in shape, 15 side leg lifts might exhaust your thigh muscles. Eventually you'll be doing 15, 30, even 60 with ease, but nothing's happening. Try those leg lifts with 1- or 2-pound ankle weights and see how that changes the exercise!

Likewise, let's say you're trying to tone that flabby underarm. One way to work that area (called the triceps), is to sit up straight on a chair or bench, raise one arm up close to the head, then slowly bend at the elbow as if you're trying to touch the back of your shoulder, keeping the upper arm and elbow close to the head. Straighten and bend the arm a few more times, always slowly and with control. Now try the same exercise holding a light weight (1-3 pounds) in your hand. See how it intensifies the work?

Beauty—Not Beef

Before you start thinking that strength training will give you a body like the body builders, let's first clear up a few stereotypes.

We've all seen the muscle men and women in magazines.

You won't become one of them. Strength training isn't about having biceps that pop your sleeves. It isn't about spending you day in the gym. It's about adding resistance work to your regular exercise routine so that you receive the physical and mental benefits of getting strong and great.

Moreover, realize that those tough, muscular models are competitors. They have the genetic makeup that allows them to develop huge muscles. Plus, they spend most of the day in rigorous training, lifting weights heavier than you'll ever attempt. (Some of them, unfortunately, also use steroids, drugs that increase muscle size, often with disastrous physical and emotional side effects.)

We promise: you will not bulk up with this program. We're not going to send you to the gym for hours of "no-pain-no-gain." You won't have to cut open your sleeves to make room for your arms. Women: your strength training won't make you look masculine. Quite the contrary, it will help you shape and accentuate those feminine curves.

The kind of strength training we recommend is slow and moderate in intensity. It builds strength, makes you look leaner, and revs up your metabolic engine.

And here's the trump card: the more muscle you have, the faster your body burns calories—even at rest! In other words, you can speed up your metabolic rate by increasing your muscle mass with a consistent strength training program. That will make it easier to eat normally and not gain body fat.

Lean Looks Good

The super skinny look is out, thank goodness. The strong, shapely, toned look is in. You're already on the right track with your aerobic exercise program. Strength training takes up where aerobic exercise quits, helping you reshape and firm your body. Strength training plus aerobic exercise are the perfect combination for balanced fitness.

Strength training helps you look and feel younger. Muscle also looks slimmer and firmer than body fat. It makes your body look tight, toned, and sculpted.

Getting Older, Getting Better

Most men and women should worry about having too little muscle, rather than too much, say the experts. This is especially important as we age. Most adults lose about one pound of muscle every two years after they reach the mid-thirties unless they do some form of strength training. Since most of us weigh more, not less, than we did at 20, we've replaced those lost muscle pounds with fat pounds. Even if we weigh the same (and how many of us do?), our lean/fat proportion has changed.

Strength training, then, is important for more than weight control and good looks. Physical activity with a strength training component is the best defense we have against the muscle loss that otherwise accompanies aging. We don't have to get frail later if we take steps now.

Reducing The Risk of Osteoporosis

Another important benefit of strength training is the protection you receive against osteoporosis. Osteoporosis is a disease that results from loss of bone. It affects one in three women over the age of 70. People tend to become less and less active as they age, and that may be the cause or at least a major contributing factor, in the development of osteopororis.

Fortunately, exercise can help head off this sometimes debilitating disease. According to the National Exercise For Life Institute, mechanical force, through gravity and pull of muscles, is the only factor known to increase bone mass and strength. "Exercise may be the most effective way to prevent age-related osteoporosis," according to Jeff Zwiefel, M.S., exercise physiologist for the Institute. "Muscle development aids in the mineralization of bone," he said, "helping bones become denser."

So don't resign yourself to getting weaker with the years—get stronger instead. Moreover, you can't stop your skin from losing elasticity as you age, but toned muscles fill up previously sagging skin to give your body a tight, shapely look. As you lose fat through your low-fat eating and exercise program, your skin will fill out with firm muscle definition. Even your posture improves with strength training, and you feel strong and confident.

Strength Training Is Easy!

You can strength train with free weights, also called dumbbells (one weight held in each hand) and barbells (a bar with weights at both ends, held by both hands). Though the commercial free weights are easy to use, you can improvise with cans of soup or plastic jugs of water. You can also use resistance machines, available in most health clubs, where you adjust the weight on the machine, then perform the movement.

For home workouts, equipment such as a Nordic Fitness Chair can give you a safe, varied, beginning weight training program, even while you're sitting comfortably watching television or conversing with the family. (This book, in fact, was written sitting on "The Chair" with the author taking frequent "fitness breaks"!) Other options include exercise-weight rubber bands, surgical tubing, or other devices that resist your movements.

Exercises Using Machines
And Free Weights

When done properly, resistance training is undoubtedly the most effective kind of strength exercise. Fitness training has an advantage over calisthenics because the overload can be adjusted more easily as strength increases.

Use trial and error to determine the amount of resistance that's right for you. Naturally, you'll be able to apply more resistance with the larger muscles of the legs and back than with the smaller arm, chest, and shoulder muscles.

Find a resistance or weight that you can do no more than 8 to 12 repetitions and perform a minimum of two sets of each exercise. When you can do 12 repetitions for two sets, add enough resistance next time to bring you back to 8 repetitions. Continue with that level of resistance until you can perform 12 repetitions, then increase the resistance in the next workout.

Generally, the heaviest resistance you can do for 8 to 12 repetitions represents approximately 75 percent of your maximum lift (the maximum weight that you can lift one time) which is ideal for developing muscle definition, strength and muscle endurance.

Getting Started

We're not asking for much of your time: just 20-30 minutes, two to three times a week. In return, you'll develop a lean, tight, well-defined look. You'll be stronger and more aware of your body's marvelous possibilities. And your fat-burning furnace will burn with a higher flame.

If you join a health club for strength training, investigate the credentials of the instructors, who should be certified by a professional fitness organization. Find out if personal training appointments are available, so you're sure to receive enough individual attention to learn the correct form and technique.

Starting Your In-Home
Strength Training Program

Busy careers and new lifestyles have created a burgeoning new trend toward at-home strength training programs. And with a balanced fitness program, you'll decrease your body's fat tissue and increase lean muscle tissue, resulting in an improved body composition.

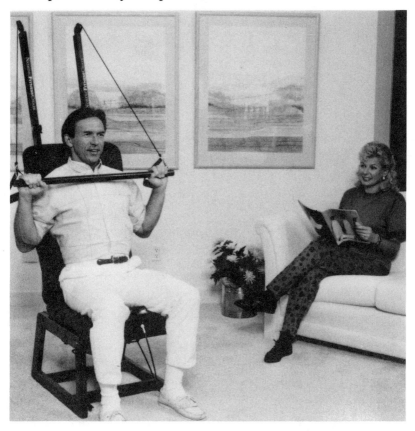

Many overweight men and women are finding that strength training helps them lose weight and improve the quality of their lives. The Nordic Fitness Chair, for example, is a convenient way to build strength and calorie-burning muscle. It takes a minimum of 10 minutes, three times a week at home or office. (Photo courtesy of NordicTrack)

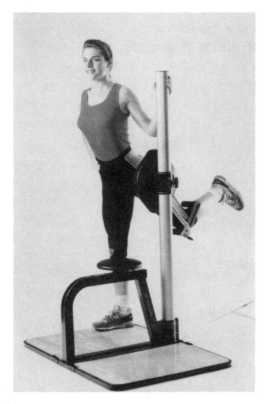

The NordicPower Plus is a convenient way to increase upper- and lower-body strength and endurance.   It's an effective way to lose weight and improve appearance because it builds the lean muscle mass that improves metabolism and tones muscles. (Photo courtesy of NordicTrack)

Staying Safe

The two keys to safety in strength training are control and technique.   Control means that you perform each move slowly, with full attention, and without momentum. You never fling your weight or throw your whole body into the move. Concentrate on the muscle you're working.   Keep the amount of weight manageable so that you can complete the move with full control.

Technique means that you understand the proper form for

each exercise. If you're learning from an instruction book or videotape, concentrate on imitating the whole body alignment, not just the limbs in motion. Look at how the back, neck and head are aligned. Are the knees bent? How much? Which body parts move? How far? How is the ending position different from the beginning? Practice without weights until you understand the form.

Tips For Effective Strength Training

1. Warm up the muscles you're going to use without weights at first. Get the muscles and joints in motion with rhythmic movement, going through each group you plan to work. Or do 10 minutes of an all-purpose exercise that warms up all your muscles for you.

2. Work through all the major muscle groups, with a total of at least 8-10 different exercises each session. Don't just do your favorites. Chances are those muscles are already your strongest. Instead, put extra time into weaker muscles, particularly the ones you don't use much in your daily life.

3. Always perform your movements slowly. The aim isn't to get to the end of a move, but rather to feel the move every inch of the way. Return to your starting position even more slowly. Don't shorten the move or just do the part that's easy.

4. Breathe! Exhale on the lifting or pulling phase, inhale when lowering or releasing. Don't hold your breath.

5. Don't overdo it. Better to do a little less than too much, especially when you're first learning your limits. Overdoing it leads to pain, discouragement, and even

injury. Mild soreness the next day—a slight ache or stiffness—is okay. It just means your muscles are adapting. It will pass as you get stronger. But if you're feeling pain that interferes with your day, you've overdone it.

6. Pay particular attention to old injury sites. Test an injured area with no weight or light weight. If there's any pain, stop. Those areas might not be as strong as before, even though you think they're completely healed. Get medical advice about rehabilitation exercises if you find you have these weak or sensitive spots.

7. Stay in tune with your body at all times. If a movement hurts, don't do it. Period.

8. Log your workouts. Keep track of the muscle groups worked, the amount of weight and number of repetitions (called "reps") for each one. You'll be surprised at how quickly you progress.

9. Increase weights slowly and not until you can do 12 reps in slow, controlled, proper form. Then, increase the weight or resistance slightly so that you can do only 6-8 reps.

10. Stretch each muscle group when you're done. If you don't stretch, you leave your muscles contracted, often resulting in soreness the next day and a decrease in flexibility over time.

11. Strength train regularly, but no more than two to three times a week. Your muscles need 48 hours to recover from intense work and to get stronger. Fill in those alternate days with aerobic exercise.

11

Choosing The Exercise Program That's Right For You

It's vital, not just important. It's vital that you reach and maintain your physical potential. It absolutely will add so much to your life.

—**David Brenner, comedian, speaking seriously about exercise**

You think you hate to exercise? You scream that you'd rather have gum surgery than work out? You'd prefer a tax audit to a gym membership?

Relax. Let go of those preconceptions of what an exercise program will be like. If you follow the suggestions in this book, you'll not only get an exercise routine going that will help you meet your fat-burning goals—but you'll create one that you'll honestly enjoy! Let's find out what kind of exercise you'll look forward to doing.

Choosing Your Activity

We'll bet you don't really hate exercise—you hate the exercise programs you've tried in the past. You're more likely to stick with a program if you can find one that suits you personally. As simple as that seems, many people don't take their own personalities and pleasures into account when setting up an exercise routine. They pick the first program that comes to mind, or the exercise they used to do, or the workout their friend does—whether or not this activity really fits them. No wonder they're counting the minutes till quitting time!

"How much choice do I have," you may ask, "when you just told me I have to have aerobics, strength training, and flexibility?" Plenty of choice. Look at the aerobic activity chart on page 111. You've got 27 choices, from basketball to square dancing. And those are just 27 of the most common aerobic activities!

Likewise, you have some choice in strength training. You need some weight or resistance to work your muscles, but you can be creative here, too. There are some terrific videotapes that teach you how to use wide latex bands (usually included with the videotape), surgical tubing, or even household items.

Your Turn: Exercising For Pleasure

To find a selection of exercise choices that will bring you more pleasure than pain, look at your personality and social preferences as well as your fitness goals. Ask yourself these questions before you choose your activities:

1. Do you want to exercise alone, or would you enjoy the company of others?

2. Do you prefer exercising indoors or outdoors?

3. Are you motivated by competition?

4. Do you like physical challenges? Risks?

5. Do you like being in control, or would you prefer a class setting?

6. Are you happier following one routine for a set period of time, or do you need the variety of a constantly changing program?

7. Do you have the self-discipline to follow an independent workout, or do you need a structured program?

8. Do you want exercise that demands mind concentration? Or would you prefer not to have to think?

9. Does music motivate you to get your body moving, or do you prefer silence?

10. Would an instructor help motivate you? If so, what personality and teaching style would motivate you best?

Analyzing Your Preferences

Now that you've made some notes about your preferences, let's see how these apply to your exercise choices. If you prefer exercising alone and outdoors, consider activities that let you enjoy the scenery and your own company—like cycling, brisk walking, running or hiking. You can involve a buddy or a group in these activities if you want outdoor exercise with others, or choose an outdoor team or group sport. Fine tune your preferences by examining whether competition or risk appeals to you.

Do you prefer exercising indoors with others? Consider trying a club or class. Clubs offer a variety of aerobics and specialty classes with strength training and flexibility segments built in—a good way to get all your fitness components in one package. They also have resistance machines, free weights, and usually high quality cardiovascular machines to give you a potpourri of choices for keeping your workout interesting. They also have a staff of fitness professionals to instruct and guide you.

If a club doesn't appeal to you, the local YMCA or community center offers individual classes, often including aerobics, martial arts, yoga, ballroom dancing, and swimming. Look at your other answers to help you pin down one or two types of classes to start.

A side benefit of joining a club or class is getting to know other people who have the same fitness goals you do. Best of all, you'll join them in experiencing how much fun exercise can be!

Are you a solo indoor exerciser by choice? You can work out with an exercise celebrity on early morning television, dance to the radio, run up and down stairs, or get an invigorating workout on a well-chosen piece of high quality indoor equipment. Sturdy indoor equipment—such as a cross-country ski exercise machine, exercise bike, rowing machine or treadmill—can keep you motivated and help you reach your goals. Think of the convenience! You can exercise any hour of the day or night. You can watch TV, talk to your family, or mentally rehearse the next day's office presentation as you work out.

Whatever your goals or present fitness level, you can find a workout that works—and you can achieve it all in the privacy of your living room.

Exercise Videotapes

What about exercise videotapes? Will they do the job? Yes, as long as you're self-disciplined enough to put on your workout wear and pop the tape in the VCR on a regular basis.

Videotapes make exercising easy and convenient, and they're ready when you are. They can motivate you to keep going. You don't even need much room: space enough to take four giant steps in all directions will do. You can wear your old sweats, talk back to the instructor, take breaks whenever you please.

Variety is the spice of exercise commitment. Mix and match a few aerobic exercise videos. The variety will keep you from getting bored once you've mastered a routine, and different workouts suit varying energy levels and moods. Add a strength training video and another for stretching, and you've got a great well-rounded program.

Gain Without Pain

A lifelong fitness program doesn't have much in common with high school physical education class or basic training. It hurts less, raises your self-esteem more, and has a chance of becoming genuinely pleasurable for its own sake. For a continued and joyful commitment to fitness, control the intensity to keep exercise comfortable and pain-free. And here's the big surprise: a more moderate, realistic approach to exercise gets you in better shape than you were in high school. The key is learning how to exercise to a point that you'll want to come back and do it again the next day.

Groaning is out—grinning is in. Once you learn how to make exercise feel good while you're doing it, you'll greet the next workout with enthusiasm.

Part III

The Honest Truth

About

Motivation

12

Choosing Change
That Fits You

The only people who like change are wet babies.
—**Mikki Williams, professional speaker**

What you do with the facts and tips in this book is far more important than knowing the facts themselves. Behavior modification—a fancy term for changing the way you do things in your everyday life—is the key. It's more important than the eating plan you choose, the exercise equipment you buy, or the cooking class in which you enroll.

All those choices are important. Some are even very important. But commitment is crucial.

Unless you make an active commitment to changing your behavior, nothing else will change either. You'll just have one more weight loss book to dust, one more piece of exercise equipment in the garage, one more collection of recipes.

Sure, change can be scary. We're creatures of habit and we're comfortable with nestling into familiar, predictable behavior patterns. But what if those comfortable habits conflict with your goals and sabotage your self-image?

You can only reach a goal by turning it into an action plan: First determine what you want to achieve. Next, define the action you need to take to make it happen.

But here's the good news: this kind of change is exciting. Think of it as traveling toward your rewards and away from the habits that drag you down. Let it be a liberating journey.

Still nervous about choosing change? Talk to friends who have made permanent lifestyle changes for health reasons. Ask how those changes have enriched their lives, rather than deprived them of habits they enjoyed. Listen to an ex-smoker talk about how much better food tastes. Hear how an avid exerciser has more energy and an improved quality of life. Let a former yo-yo dieter tell you how much better she likes herself now.

If you're a little wary now, that's normal. You're used to a certain way of living, eating, relating to others, and simply getting through the day. The "you" of six months from now could be very different.

This is a voyage, and the direction is clearly and honestly marked. It isn't a military march. You won't always be in step. And you won't go at the same pace as anyone else. You might take a few side trips before you reach your destination. You might hit a few rocks and boulders, a roadblock and even a volcano or two.

But you'll go on and eventually get there. When you look back, you'll be glad you chose change.

Making Important Changes

This book is not about making sweeping changes in your eating and activity habits all at once. You've tried that in the past and it didn't work. At best, it felt uncomfortable, like wearing someone else's clothes, not your size, style, or personal choice. At worst, it felt like prison, a state of continual deprivation. You couldn't wait to shed the restrictions and break out.

Here is the alternative to drastic change: Make small, important changes that you can live with comfortably, even pleasurably. Make choices and changes gradually.

If you're considering changing your clothing style, for example, you don't throw out everything in your closet and buy all new outfits. You start by choosing one new item or ensemble that fits well, looks good, and makes you want to wear it. You see how it suits your lifestyle. If you like the way it looks and feels, you gradually incorporate that style into more outfits. Little by little, you phase out the old and bring in the new.

Commit yourself to a six-month program of small, important changes. Visualize where you want to be in six months, and dedicate the time to get there. Make a six-month commitment to the new person you want to become.

By the time a half-year rolls by, your new changes will have become comfortable habits. Oh sure, you'll discard some that don't fit and you'll substitute others. But you'll emerge with a new set of habits that fits you and suits your style. And best of all, you'll have them for life.

The results you want are within your reach—so reach out your arms and grab them!

Changing For Life

> *You can't help getting older.*
> *But you don't have to get old!*
> **—George Burns, comedian**

What's the biggest reason for making lifestyle changes? What's the ultimate aim, the big picture, the mission? No, not just weight loss. It's quality of life. You want to improve your vitality and health not just for six months, not just for this decade, but for life. You want to be spritely and strong for the rest of your years. You want your body to function with power and independence as you get older. You want your life to get more full with each birthday, not more limited.

Here's what we mean: Jake, 87, started exercising this year when a local health club started a seniors' class. "My body isn't unhealthy," he told his instructor, "just neglected." And within 30 days his fitness blossomed in concert with his enjoyment of his new-found abilities. He likes the class because the focus is on functional exercises that improve his stamina, balance and flexibility. Plus, he has discovered that moving to music can be fun. He attends his meetings faithfully three times a week and has asked about exercises he can do at home on the other days.

See what we mean? Exercise is fun! But to make it so, you've got to shift your attitude from thinking that losing weight is the most important goal in your life. Look beyond weight loss to the other parts of your life you want to improve. You have the power to create changes in your life, not just in your waistline.

Once you start looking at yourself and what you really want, you may find yourself making other changes. You may get a new hairstyle, change the furniture, or ask for a job reassignment. You might even discover that you like change!

Your Turn: Looking At Your Habits

The information you've learned here has helped you understand more about your body, gain a new perspective on your personal weight history, and reevaluate your weight loss goals. Now it's time to pull together the issues you defined as most important and immediate to you, and begin changing yourself.

Information can empower you and other people's stories can inspire you. But only YOU can motivate yourself to make those choices that will lead to your personal goals. Grab your pencil again and tie all this information together.

1. List the habits you have that might be stopping you from losing weight:

2. Which of these habits were due to lack of information and will be easy to change now that you know better?

3. Which of these habits will be harder to change?

4. Decide you will work on changing one small habit each week and one large habit each month. Choose the habits you want to change first, and put them in the order you will work on them:

13

Motivation:
Making This Book
Work For You

Be sure to keep a mirror always nigh
In some convenient, handy sort of place,
And now and then look squarely in thine eye,
with thyself keep ever face to face.

—John Kendrick Bangs (1862-1922)

You can reach goals if you really want to, but it isn't enough to just want the results. You must actively pursue those results, to do whatever it takes to get there, and to keep on doing it. Determination plus action equals success.

Are You Determined Enough?

You've known people who are all talk and no action. Maybe you used to be one of those. Anyone can talk a good line about wanting to change. We're asking you to put your muscle where your mouth is.

That means shaking your head from side to side when someone offers you fatty foods. It means pushing yourself away from the table when you're no longer physically hungry. And it means finding exercise activities that you truly enjoy, so that you'll look forward to doing them. You must set goals that you want with all your heart, mind and body so much that you'll go after your goals with whatever it takes.

Remember when you got your first bicycle or pair of skates? How long did it take to learn how to balance? To control your direction and speed? How many times did you fall down?

Learning the skills that made your goal a reality wasn't fun at first, but "give up" wasn't in your vocabulary. You kept getting up and trying again. Your goal was strong and clear, and you wanted it. You believed in your power to reach your goal, which was crucial to your success. You were determined, despite skinned knees and Mom's gasps each time you took a spill, despite the older kids' taunts. Remember?

Recapture that degree of determination. You need to reassess your goals and put them in a form that makes you say, "Yes, I want to do this, and I can do it. I'm starting NOW."

Big Goals, Smaller Goals, And Resolutions

At the beginning of this book, we asked you to consider your reasons for reading it. You probably answered, "I want to lose weight," or maybe, "I want to lose (choose one: 20, 40, 60) pounds by Christmas." Now that you're more knowledgeable, you'll probably revise your answer and name these new, long-term goals:

Big Goals:
- I want to lose body fat and keep it off.
- I want to avoid the dieting/regaining cycle.
- I want to feel healthy and energetic.
- I want to look my best.

You know how to reach these goals. You've learned from this book that accomplishing your goals depends on making a series of changes and actively pursuing them. It will be easier to reach your goals if you first turn those Big Goals into Smaller Goals, such as these:

Smaller Goals:

- I'll decrease the amount of fat I eat.
- I'll stop eating when I'm no longer hungry.
- I'll adopt a balanced fitness program including regular aerobic exercise and strength training.
- I'll find physical activities I enjoy enough to make them part of my daily life.

Now let's break those Smaller Goals into more manageable parts, or Resolutions, that put you in control of meeting your goals. Here are some samples to start you thinking. Of course, you will have to define your own needs and your own resolutions.

Sample Resolutions

- ✓ I'll get my body fat tested and take my measurements to see where I am now.
- ✓ I'll get rid of the ice cream, fudge and other tempting foods in the house.
- ✓ I'll get a low-fat, whole foods cookbook and try one new recipe a week in place of a high-fat meal. (Remember to double the recipe and freeze the leftovers to use when you're too tired to cook.)
- ✓ When we go out for pizza, I'll fill my plate at the salad bar and just have two slices of pizza instead of my usual.

✓ I'll phone one of the companies that sell in-home exercise equipment and ask for the free information.

✓ I'll borrow a friend's bicycle this weekend and see if I still enjoy cycling as much as I used to. If I do, I'll look in the Sunday paper for used bikes for sale.

✓ I'll rent a different exercise videotape each week and see which one I like well enough to buy.

✓ I'll walk instead of drive for short errands.

✓ I'll take the kids hiking on weekends in nice weather.

What's different about the Big Goals, Small Goals and Resolutions method? You're formulating personally meaningful goals and setting up an active plan to reach them. Your goals become attainable because they rely solely on your own actions—not on luck, other people, or magic. Your Resolutions are specific and manageable enough that you can see your success day by day. Your own behavior puts the Smaller Goals under your control. Step by step, the Big Goals get closer. You are proving to yourself that you have the power to make your dreams a reality!

Positive Goal Setting

In the following section, you'll be asked to redefine your goals. You're going to set your Big Goals, then break them down into Smaller Goals, then into Resolutions, like the samples above. Make your goals:

- positive, not negative
- active, not passive

- realistic
- flexible
- manageable
- personal behavioral changes
- compatible with the way you live
- health-giving
- lifelong behavioral changes.

These suggestions might seem simplistic. You might even be tempted to skip this part and just start your program. But think back: how many times have you set New Year's Resolutions only to abandon them before January 15? How many times have you vowed, "This time I'll really do it!"—whatever "it" was at the time—and then failed to achieve your goal?

Now, think of a goal that you have achieved. Remember passing an important exam, making the team or the school play, getting an important job, buying your first house?

Whichever accomplishment was yours, how did you do it? Did you prepare for it? Did you figure out exactly what steps you'd have to follow to get there? Did you have a plan? Were you motivated to do whatever it took? Of course.

Your Turn: Defining Your Goals

Here, or in your private notebook, define the Big Goals, and then define the Smaller Goals and Resolutions that will guide you to accomplish your Big Goals. Be careful to make your goals active, specific, and personal. Make them fit you and the way you live. Be sure you can take charge of meeting these goals.

Every few weeks, reassess these goals. Change them or add to them if you see ways to ensure success more fully.

Goals are living and mobile. They can guide you only if they reflect the person you are. And they reflect the person you are becoming.

BIG GOALS

(1)_____

(2)_____

SMALLER GOALS

(1)_____

(2)_____

(3)_____

(4)_____

RESOLUTIONS

(1)_____

(2)_____

(3)_____

(4)_____

BIG GOALS

(1)_____

(2)_____

SMALLER GOALS

(1)_____

(2)_____

(3)_____

(4)_____

(5)_____

RESOLUTIONS

(1)_____

(2)_____

(3)_____

(4)_____

(5)_____

14

Getting Started

We know what we are,
but know not what we may be.

—William Shakespeare, in *Hamlet*

It's up to you now. You've got the facts, you've set your
goals, and now it's time to start your action plan. You know
what to do, and you understand the reasons for your choices.

Of course, knowing what and why isn't the same as
knowing how. Putting these changes into action isn't easy.
It's a leap, more than a step.

You've probably started many times. Starting is easy.
Your motivation is high, your excitement spurs you on. But
keeping these changes in your life day after day, week after
week, can be a struggle until your mind and body adapt to your
new way of living. Make it easier by creating an action plan
that fits you personally—one that feels like a healthful vaca-
tion, not a jail sentence.

Your Turn: Looking At Your Stumbling Blocks

Throughout the earlier chapters, you've written the answers to questions about your self-image, weight history, diet

history, exercise history, eating habits, and goals and resolutions. You've chosen the changes you want to make. Now let's take an honest look at some stumbling blocks that might get in your way.

Take a few minutes now and read through your earlier answers. As you do this, write down all the reasons, excuses, and other obstacles that can prevent you from making the changes you've chosen. Include both internal and external stumbling blocks. For example, an internal block might be, "I can't control my eating when I'm tired. I eat everything in sight after 7 p.m." An external block might be, "The vending machine at work has only high-calorie, high-fat snacks" or "The kids insist on dessert every night."

WHAT ARE YOUR STUMBLING BLOCKS?	
Internal	External

Case Study: Kent

Kent, 39, tried to start exercising dozens of times. He tried aerobics classes, but felt frozen in the midst of a moving sea of coordinated people, mostly women. He tried a gym, but was put off by the competitive attitude of the men. His stumbling blocks were his feelings of inadequacy and his fears of being judged by more competent athletes. "I was a nerd in high school, never a jock. The whole gym scene made me uncomfortable. It still does. I still hate locker rooms!"

Then Kent saw a TV commercial for a high-quality rowing machine and he decided to give it a whirl.

"It was the greatest thing I could have done," Kent reported. "The NordicRow was perfect for me. It exercised all my major upper and lower body muscle groups and the seat design cradles my lower back so there's no strain. It's fully adjustable so as I got stronger and more fit, the NordicRow 'kept up' with me.

"Best of all, I can do this exercise right in my home, without worrying about other people judging my athletic abilities. It's terrific."

Personalize Your Plan

There are plenty of personal exercise plans you can put together. Just make sure the plan fits your lifestyle as well as your fitness level. Look at the attractions of different types and styles of exercise.

If you work indoors all day and long to be outside, for example, a daily outdoor activity will feel like a treat. If you like to dance to the radio but would feel embarrassed by other people watching you, an aerobics videotape might suit you better. If you want to spend your free time with the family, choose an activity you can do with them, such as bicycling, or a home exercise, such as a rower or ski machine.

Examine your likes, dislikes, joys and fears, and choose activities that feel comfortable and inviting. This will do more to ensure your success than the most expensive pair of jogging shoes or a membership to the classiest health club. Once you get used to regular exercise, you might find, as Kent did, that you're ready to branch out and try new experiences. But start with an activity that feels right, and let it become a habit.

Personalize your eating plan as well as your exercise plan. If you're constantly on the go, you'll need ways to eat right without many extra hours of preparation. If you eat out at lunchtime, you'll want to sleuth nearby restaurants ahead of time to find the best low-fat offerings.

Keep your goals and resolutions in your mind and in your view. Post them on the refrigerator at home and inside your desk drawer at work. Keep a copy in the car. Go public: tell your friends and family about the changes you're actively making, and enlist their help. Maybe they'd like to set their own goals and resolutions and join you.

Case Study: Ginnie and Phyllis

Ginnie, 33, gained 10 pounds last year. She kept starting to exercise, but couldn't get herself to make it a habit. When she learned that her sister-in-law, Phyllis, faced the same problem, they decided to exercise together.

Phyllis wanted to run or bicycle, though, and Ginnie wanted to do aerobic dancing. They tried each other's choices, but still preferred their own.

They finally agreed to meet at Jazzercise four times a week. Then Phyllis would go off to run or bicycle for an hour, while Ginnie took the class. They would meet again after class and compare notes about how their programs were going.

Ginnie and Phyllis are now in their third month of being

exercise buddies. "Just knowing that Phyllis counts on me to meet her gets me there every time," says Ginnie. "We agreed not to cancel except in extreme emergency, like a broken leg or the house on fire. If the weather's bad, Phyllis does the class with me. If I'm low on energy, maybe I'll just walk instead of doing the class. But I always get there, and I always do something."

Phyllis is just as enthusiastic. She admits she was luke-warm about the idea at first. "I've always been a loner. I like to run and bike ride because I can get away from people, and I don't have to talk to anyone or make compromises. But it got too easy to make excuses. Now that I have to meet Ginnie, I plan my schedule around that exercise date. And you know what? Jazzercise is kind of fun!"

A Buddy In Need Is A Buddy Indeed

The buddy system is one of the best ways to stay on track. Team up with a pal. Share goals and resolutions. Make exercise appointments, as Ginnie and Phyllis do. Research healthy foods together. Go grocery shopping and cook together once a week. Try each other's pet exercise. Explore an activity new to both of you.

Use your buddy for psychological support, too. Remember those evenings when you filled the second bowl of ice cream, grabbed the whole bag of Oreos, and turned your back on your resolutions? Remember the visit to your mother, when she nagged you about your weight, while piling food on your plate? How about the time you stared at the leftover birthday cake and told yourself, "No, I won't . . . I won't . . . Oh—what the heck."

A buddy is someone you can call for a quick shot of willpower. Your buddy can help talk you out of self-defeating behavior, and you can do the same for her or him. It takes honesty to ask for help in this. But if you tend to eat compulsively and destructively, you might need help to get past those pivotal moments. If a buddy isn't enough, or if you don't dare ask someone for help, try one of the organized support groups you'll find on our earlier chart.

Where do you find a buddy? Ask your family, friends, neighbors, or co-workers. Then widen your circle: consider the parents of your children's friends, members of any church or social group you frequent. Mention your plan at parties and family gatherings.

Look in the newspaper for listings of outdoor activity groups. Whether or not you enjoy group activities, you'll meet other people interested in being fit.

Sometimes buddies emerge from exercise activities, instead of the other way around. If you take a class, go to the gym or walk the park at a certain time of day, notice which other people are frequently there when you are. Smile and nod when you pass them, and if they seem friendly, say a few words.

Next time, you might ask them a question about their exercise activity, or mention that you see them often, and you wonder how they stick to their program so easily. Be aware that many people like to stay with their own thoughts while exercising, or they might be nervous about strangers striking up conversations. If they don't want to talk, respect that and don't take it personally. But many people will be pleased to talk about themselves and flattered that you asked. You'll get some helpful tips, and maybe a buddy.

A System Of Rewards

You might want to establish an on-going rewards system to keep yourself motivated. The ultimate rewards—improved health, fitness and appearance—might take a while to show themselves. Meanwhile, you might stick to your weight loss or exercise program more easily if you create a system of short-term rewards along the way.

Try filling a jar with the money you save each time you "just say no" to one of your fattening habits. Just drop the money saved in the jar. Each time you walk or bicycle instead of drive, put gas money in the jar.

Or decide on a small sum of money that you'll drop in the jar when you exercise. Make it small enough that you won't make your kids go barefoot to support your jar, but large enough to be meaningful.

Then when your jar is full, give yourself a reward. Don't use it for daily expenses or something ordinary. Don't spend it on someone else. Indulge yourself. Buy yourself something special, something you probably would never have bought for yourself.

Caution: make this a non-food reward. Taking yourself out to dinner, for example, will reinforce an idea you're trying to eliminate: that food is a reward. Instead, promise yourself presents that will keep you more firmly focused on your weight loss success: new exercise clothes or equipment, or music for your workout. Or give yourself a stress release gift, like a baby-sitter for the afternoon or a massage.

You'll get other rewards, too, and they won't cost you the money in your jar. As soon as you start cutting down your dietary fat and increasing your exercise frequency, you'll start feeling results in your mind and body. You'll have more energy, more self-esteem, and less stress. You'll feel powerful, in control of your decisions. And—if you've personalized your plan effectively—you'll start to enjoy the process of change.

Your Personal Action Plan

Action time! Look over your Big Goals, Smaller Goals and Resolutions, examine the stumbling blocks you'll need to deal with, and set up your personal action plan to bring your goals to life. Do this for one week at a time.

Include in your plan some very simple changes that you'll have very little trouble accomplishing next week, such as these:

- I'll carry a calculator to the supermarket so I can look for foods under 30 percent fat.
- I'll buy a low-fat cookbook.
- I'll take my measurements.
- I'll investigate in-home exercise equipment.

Include at least one substantial change each week. By "substantial," we don't mean drastic or radical. We mean a change that will make a noticeable contribution towards helping you reach your goal. Here are a few examples:

- I'll walk for 20 minutes on Tuesday, Thursday and Saturday.
- I'll cook two meals from my new low-fat cookbook.

And here's a tip: include in your action plan a "contingency plan" in case you can't (or won't) do what you planned. For example, if you resolve to walk, include what you'll do in case of rain (e.g. exercise indoors with a rower or ski machine). If you plan to eat only low-fat foods at dinner, include what you'll do at a restaurant. Think of where you personally get trapped, and plan your escape route. Ready? Get set, go!

MY ACTION PLAN

WEEK 1

_____

_____

_____

_____

_____

WEEK 2

_____

_____

_____

_____

WEEK 3

_____

_____

_____

_____

MY ACTION PLAN

WEEK 4

_____

_____

_____

_____

_____

WEEK 5

_____

_____

_____

_____

_____

WEEK 6

_____

_____

_____

_____

15

Putting It
All Together

Whatever you're going to be,
you're becoming now.

—Noah J. Kassman, M.D., to his daughter
(who grew up to write this book)

Charting Your Progress

Now it's up to you. You've got the facts. You've set your
goals. You've got your action plan. It's time to start. Use
these pages to record and chart your progress, or, if you prefer,
photocopy them to keep in your private notebook. Make extra
copies when you're about to run out.

Use Photographs

Get a friend to help you, and start by recording your
"before" information. Dress in swim wear or other revealing,
hide-no-flaws clothing, and have your friend take a series of
photographs.

Use bright lighting. Take photos from the front, the side,
the rear. Take both whole-body shots and close-ups. Pose!

Pretend you're a fashion model, movie star, or body builder. Decorate yourself with hats, jewelry, feathers, whatever amuses you. Laugh a lot. Make it fun to get the best, worst, and wildest pictures of the body you have today.

See? You're enjoying your body more already. You don't need to hate your fat to lose it. In fact, the more you like yourself, the easier time you'll have progressing toward your goals. Honest!

After you get the film developed and your photos printed, choose two to mount in the pages following this section. Choose the one you like the best and get it enlarged. Keep the ones you don't like; they're part of the record of your journey. Call them, "Before."

Every four to six months, take another series of photographs. Wear the same clothes (until they're too loose to wear any more) and, again, ham it up. Try to imitate the same poses, so that you can see your body's changes clearly by comparing photos from different dates.

Once you're making visible progress, you can motivate yourself to stick with your program by putting a series of photos on the mirror or refrigerator.

Record Your Measurements

If you decide to get your body fat tested, record your results. Otherwise, record your measurements as the simplest way to see how much fat you're losing and how you're reshaping your body.

You'll get more accurate measurements if you get a friend to help you. The accuracy of self-measurements suffers because you have to twist and contort to position the tape measure and read it. Stand up straight, but naturally. Don't distort the measurements by sucking in your belly or clenching your buttocks!

Every few weeks, take your measurements again. Women, skip your premenstrual or menstrual times if you tend to bloat.

We've included a space to record scale weight because you'll probably want to see how your pound loss compares to your inches lost. But don't lose sight of the fact that inches lost are more important than pounds lost. Remember, you lose inches with body fat loss.

Date_____
Bust/Chest_____
Belly*_____
Waist_____
Hips (at hip bone)_____
Buttocks*_____
Thigh*_____
Upper arm_____
Neck_____
Scale weight (optional)_____

Date_____
Bust/Chest_____
Belly*_____
Waist_____
Hips (at hip bone)_____
Buttocks*_____
Thigh*_____
Upper arm_____
Neck_____
Scale weight (optional)_____

Date_____
Bust/Chest_____
Belly*_____
Waist_____
Hips (at hip bone)_____
Buttocks*_____
Thigh*_____
Upper arm_____
Neck_____
Scale weight (optional)_____

Date_____
Bust/Chest_____
Belly*_____
Waist_____
Hips (at hip bone)_____
Buttocks*_____
Thigh*_____
Upper arm_____
Neck_____
Scale weight (optional)_____

*Take the belly, buttocks and thigh measurements at the widest point of your body.

PHOTO 1: "BEFORE"

DATE:_____

Bust/Chest_____

Belly*_____

Waist_____

Hips (at hip bone)_____

Buttocks*_____

Thigh*_____

Upper arm_____

Neck_____

Scale weight (optional)_____

*Take the belly, buttocks and thigh measurements at the widest point of your body.

PHOTO 2: "AFTER"

DATE:_____

Bust/Chest_____

Belly*_____

Waist_____

Hips (at hip bone)_____

Buttocks*_____

Thigh*_____

Upper arm_____

Neck_____

Scale weight (optional)_____

*Take the belly, buttocks and thigh measurements at the widest point of your body.

Your Eating Record

Each day, give your eating a "report card" by grading it "A" to "F" according to this scale:

A= Low in fat (under 30 percent), high in complex carbohydrates, moderate in protein, moderate in amount, low in empty calories. If you could eat like this all the time, you wouldn't have a problem!

B= Almost an A, except you ate slightly more than you needed. Still, it was all good, healthful food.

C= Not too bad, but not good enough to help you reach your goals. You ate more fat than you needed, and maybe skipped the salad, but you didn't really overeat. This is better than the "old days," but not what you were aiming for. Your choices will be better tomorrow.

D= Oops. You ate more than you needed, and you'd be embarrassed to list your foods here. You wish you hadn't done it, and you'll try to avoid doing it again. You'll aim for an A or B tomorrow.

F= You derailed. The train is off the track. Your eating got out of control. You're ready to give up. Wait, it was just one day. It's over. Get back on track again. Read your goals, your action plan. Write about today in your private notebook. Decide that tomorrow will be a new beginning.

Note: If you're having a D or F day, and you catch yourself before the day is over and get back on track, raise yourself one grade. See, the day wasn't a total loss after all!

EATING RECORD EVALUATION

WEEK 1:

DATE	GRADE	COMMENTS
Sunday		
Monday		
Tuesday		
Wednesday		
Thursday		
Friday		
Saturday		

WEEK 2:

DATE	GRADE	COMMENTS
Sunday		
Monday		
Tuesday		
Wednesday		
Thursday		
Friday		
Saturday		

WEEK 3:

DATE	GRADE	COMMENTS
Sunday		
Monday		
Tuesday		
Wednesday		
Thursday		
Friday		
Saturday		

EATING RECORD EVALUATION

WEEK 4:

DATE	GRADE	COMMENTS
Sunday		
Monday		
Tuesday		
Wednesday		
Thursday		
Friday		
Saturday		

WEEK 5:

DATE	GRADE	COMMENTS
Sunday		
Monday		
Tuesday		
Wednesday		
Thursday		
Friday		
Saturday		

WEEK 6:

DATE	GRADE	COMMENTS
Sunday		
Monday		
Tuesday		
Wednesday		
Thursday		
Friday		
Saturday		

Your Exercise Record

Exercise is the only way to turn your body into a fat-burning machine. You can become leaner only if you're consistent in your exercise program. Keeping an exercise record will help you stay consistent. Plan to do some kind of exercise or physical activity every day, making it a habit.

When you wake up in the morning, don't ask yourself if you feel like exercising. Instead, ask yourself which exercise you feel like doing. In the last chapter, you reserved a time each day solely for physical activity, and you chose a variety of activities to do.

Each week, be sure you include three or more days of aerobic exercise, and two or more of some kind of strength training. In addition, add physical activity into your daily routine, whether it's walking to the post office, raking leaves, or washing the windows.

Each day, record your exercise and the other physical activities that you do. Write the type of exercise and the number of minutes under each appropriate category. Each week, evaluate the success of your program and comment on your enjoyment of it.

1. How many minutes of aerobic exercise did you do this week?

2. How many times did you strength train?

3. What did you enjoy most about exercising this week?

4. What progress do you see since last week?

5. What activities would you like to do next week?

WEEK 1

	Aerobic Exercise	Strength Training	Other Activity
Sunday			
Monday			
Tuesday			
Wednesday			
Thursday			
Friday			
Saturday			

WEEK 2

	Aerobic Exercise	Strength Training	Other Activity
Sunday			
Monday			
Tuesday			
Wednesday			
Thursday			
Friday			
Saturday			

WEEK 3

	Aerobic Exercise	Strength Training	Other Activity
Sunday			
Monday			
Tuesday			
Wednesday			
Thursday			
Friday			
Saturday			

WEEK 4

	Aerobic Exercise	Strength Training	Other Activity
Sunday			
Monday			
Tuesday			
Wednesday			
Thursday			
Friday			
Saturday			

WEEK 5

	Aerobic Exercise	Strength Training	Other Activity
Sunday			
Monday			
Tuesday			
Wednesday			
Thursday			
Friday			
Saturday			

WEEK 6

	Aerobic Exercise	Strength Training	Other Activity
Sunday			
Monday			
Tuesday			
Wednesday			
Thursday			
Friday			
Saturday			

Some people find it easier to stick to a program if they keep a food diary. They aren't as tempted to cheat if they know they have to write it down. If you're one of these, add a food diary to the progress pages here. You can dedicate a date book to this or use notebook pages. If you decide to do this, really do it! If you don't want it on your page, don't put it in your mouth. Each day, also fill out the Eating Record Evaluation.

Other folks find it irritating to write down every bite they eat and might abandon a program that insisted they do. This is your personalized plan. If a food diary wouldn't work for you, then just fill out the Eating Record Evaluation each day to keep you on track.

Notes

Appendix

Annotated Bibliography

This is the only weight loss book you'll ever need, but it's not the only good one out there. If this book has whetted your appetite for more information, here are some excellent resources.

Breaking the Diet Habit, Janet Polivy & C. Peter Herman, 1983, Basic Books.

Especially useful for the compulsive dieter, this book examines whether or not dieting really delivers the desired payoffs: slimness, health, happiness, and attractiveness. "What if weight loss isn't the magic key to success in all these respects?" The authors lead us to analyze what we stand to gain from weight loss or dieting, and whether we're likely to get what we want. The authors want to open the possibility of choice to dieters who have felt compelled.

The Callaway Diet: Successful Permanent Weight Control for Starvers, Stuffers, and Skippers, C. Wayne Callaway, M.D. with Catharine Whitney, 1990, Bantam.

Here, in easy, readable form, are the facts about weight and dieting, backed up with descriptions of the research studies which led to those conclusions. The second half of the book teaches former dieters how to normalize their metabolic rate. The book is aimed specifically at three types of dieters: the starver, with a long-term, repeated pattern of semi-starvation on low-calorie diets; the skipper, who eats two-thirds or more of her daily calories in the evening; and the stuffer, who overeats.

The Dieter's Dilemma: Eating Less and Weighing More, William Bennett, M.D. and Joel Gurin, 1982, Basic Books.

Upbeat, convincing arguments and perspective against dieting and for self-acceptance, health and activity. This book describes research studies on whether fat people eat more than thin (they don't), what happens when thin people try to get fat, how fat rats get if they are fed their favorite foods or deprived of food or exercise. This is a splendid reference book, written at the lay person's level, but the number of studies gets tedious, and you'll probably need to read it in small doses.

Fit or Fat?, Covert Bailey, 1977, Houghton Mifflin.

Bailey revolutionized the public's understanding of body fat, the difference between overfat and overweight, and the value of aerobic exercise for fat loss and fitness gains. This book will never be outdated, because the truths it tells are timeless. Bailey compares different types of exercise and explains why aerobic activities at moderate intensity work best. He also covers low-fat eating.

The Fit or Fat Woman, Covert Bailey and Lea Bishop, 1989, Houghton Mifflin.

This book addresses the special body fat problems common to women. Excess fat is a symptom, not the problem, says Bailey. The problem is what makes you gain fat easily. "You can decrease fat, a symptom, with dieting or with surgery, but you haven't changed your metabolism or your tendency to get fat." Aerobic exercise, body building, and balanced dieting are the keys for changing the way your body puts on and holds onto body fat, and Bailey shows you why.

Great Shape: The First Exercise Guide for Large Women, Pat Lyons, R.N. and Debby Burgard, 1988, Bull Publishing.

This unusual exercise book shouts that fat and fit are not mutually exclusive, and that physical activity is a need and a pleasure, whatever your size. This isn't a weight loss book. It's about enjoying exercise because it feels good to move, and it gives us bodies that are "more firm, sleek, strong and capable," whatever our weight. Don't put your life on hold while waiting to get thin, says this book, get moving now. This book shows you how to find the physical activity you'll enjoy.

Jane Brody's Good Food Book: Living the High-Carbohydrate Way, Jane Brody, 1985, W.W. Norton & Co.

Here's all you need to know about eating and cooking nutritiously in an excellent, comprehensive (700 pages) book. Brody doesn't suggest going to extremes. She promotes high carbohydrates, low fat, low sugar, trimming unnecessary calories, and adapting your favorite recipe or moderating your diet, rather than trying to eat entirely differently. A readable, practical resource.

Lose Weight Naturally: The No-Diet, No-Willpower Method of Successful Weight Loss, Mark Bricklin, rev. ed. 1989, Rodale Press.

A good, basic, sensible guide for taking stock of self-defeating weight loss attitudes and behavior in the past, and educating yourself about how to lose weight successfully without going on a radical diet. Includes attitudinal strategies, painless calorie cutting, how to eat out (including best choices for different types of restaurants), healthiest cooking methods, food ratings, and tips and hints to keep you on track. Perhaps too much emphasis on calorie counting, though.

Making Peace With Food: Freeing Yourself from the Diet/ Weight Obsession, Susan Kano, 1989, Harper & Row.

This self-help workbook is for people at war with their bodies and with food. If you're a chronic dieter, you'll learn ways to shake loose of your preoccupation with weight loss and your obsession with food. Kano's goal: "to help you free yourself from the diet/weight obsession." She teaches and encourages you to recognize physical hunger, overcome the fear of eating spontaneously, get physically active, and accept your own body and its setpoint.

The New Fitness Formula of the 90's, 1990, The National Exercise For Life Institute, Box 2000, Excelsior, MN 55331.

This unique collection of articles by the nation's top health writers and fitness authorities explores the importance of combining a regular program of strength training with aerobic exercise. Published by The National Exercise For Life Institute, one of the nation's foremost exercise research and information organizations. Follow the plan in this formula for balanced fitness and you'll achieve optimum health and quality of life. Fully illustrated with plenty of tips on getting the most out of exercise.

Nutrition Action Healthletter, *monthly newsletter,* Center for Science in the Public Interest, Suite 300, 1875 Connecticut Ave. N.W., Washington, DC 20009-5728.

This lively newsletter is a feisty watchdog, barking at deceptive advertising and inadequate labeling of food products, and sniffing out the latest research related to nutrition and health. A subscription is indispensable if you want to be the first on your block to learn the facts, especially those that the food industry doesn't want to tell you. You'll be a wiser shopper and a smarter eater with this newsletter.

The Strength Connection, edited by the Institute for Aerobics Research, with foreword by Kenneth Cooper, M.D., M.P.H., 1990.

This unique book has everything readers need and want from a self-help fitness book: scientific information that's easy to understand, motivational tools that you can use, and easy-to-administer fitness assessments. This innovative guide provides the important link between muscle strength and quality of life. It's a must for your fitness reading list!

Tufts University Diet & Nutrition Letter, monthly newsletter, 53 Park Place, New York, NY 10007.

You'll find in this well-respected newsletter research findings that you won't find anywhere else: what foods are consumed by prime time TV stars during the top ranked programs (answer: junk foods high in sugar and fat); whether packaging chemicals leach into foods during microwaving, and even comparisons of top-selling weight-loss programs. You'll get the latest word each month.

Tufts University Guide to Total Nutrition, Stanley Gershoff, Ph.D., 1990, Harper & Row.

This nutrition reference book is organized and presented so clearly and practically that you'll use it often. For example, the chapter "The Nutritional Shopping Cart" takes each type of food and gives the nutritional benefits, nutritional cautions, and shopping tips. You're shown how to make better choices for the foods you like, rather than being asked to give up that food. You'll learn how to read labels, nourish your children, and fight fat nutritionally, among many topics.

The Underground Shopper's Guide to Health & Fitness,
Sue Goldstein, 1987, Fawcett Columbine.

This entertaining, practical (and often funny) book is chock full (475 pages) of positive information. Reading it is like chatting with an enthusiastic pal who has lost weight the "right" way—with a low-fat, high complex carbohydrate diet—after years of trying the wrong ways. Her explanations are clear and non-technical. She lists other helpful books and resources. The long spa section might be out of date, however.

About The Author:

Joan Price, M.A., is a widely published freelance writer whose articles on health and fitness have appeared in 25 major publications. She is owner/director of Unconventional Moves, providing exercise programs for San Francisco Bay Area conventions and businesses. An IDEA Foundation-certified instructor, she teaches in two northern California health clubs and trains instructors in the LI Teknique.

Other Books From NordicPress:

- *The Strength Connection*
- *The New Fitness Formula of the 90's*